Cases in Structural Cardiac Inte

Anitha Varghese • Neal Uren • Peter Ludman
Editors

Cases in Structural Cardiac Intervention

Springer

Editors
Anitha Varghese
London
UK

Neal Uren
Royal Infirmary of Edinburgh
Edinburgh
UK

Peter Ludman
Department of Cardiology
Queen Elizabeth Hospital
Birmingham
UK

ISBN 978-1-4471-7378-6 ISBN 978-1-4471-4981-1 (eBook)
DOI 10.1007/978-1-4471-4981-1

Printed on acid-free paper

This Springer imprint is published by Springer Nature
The registered company is Springer-Verlag London Ltd.
The registered company address is: 236 Gray's Inn Road, London WC1X 8HB, United Kingdom

Contents

Contributors

Editors

Anitha Varghese, MD, MRCP London, UK

Neal Uren Royal Infirmary of Edinburgh, Edinburgh, UK

Peter F. Ludman, MA, MD, FRCP Queen Elizabeth Hospital, Birmingham, UK

Authors

Patrick Calvert Papworth Hospital NHS Foundation Trust, Papworth Everard, Cambridge, UK

Pradeep Magapu Liverpool Heart and Chest Hospital, Liverpool, UK

Nick Palmer Liverpool Heart and Chest Hospital, Liverpool, UK

Introduction

Structural heart disease intervention is a major area of development in cardiology. A desire to minimise the invasiveness of interventions and reduce patient exposure to risk have been the main drivers in developing catheter-based intervention in preference to open-heart surgery. Over the past 9 years, transcatheter aortic valve implantation (TAVI) has become the standard treatment for patients deemed inoperable or high risk for conventional aortic valve replacement, with evidence of its potential in those at intermediate risk. Mitral valve interventions are also moving forward in development. Percutaneous balloon mitral valvuloplasty (BMV) is a catheter-based technique that achieves commisurotomy in the context of pliable mitral stenosis in patients with rheumatic heart disease and has replaced surgery as the favoured approach. BMV also has an important role in patients with significant mitral stenosis during pregnancy. Percutaneous mitral valve repair encompasses several catheter-based techniques to either diminish annular dilatation or correct poor mitral valve leaflet coaptation in patients with severe mitral regurgitation at too high risk for conventional surgical mitral valve repair or replacement.

In patients who have undergone previous cardiac surgery and valve replacement, paravalvular regurgitation may occur following detachment of the surgical valve ring through stitch failure, wear and tear or after endocarditis. The risk of re-do valve replacement surgery is high and may be prohibitive, leading to a preference for an initial catheter-based strategy of plugging residual gaps external to the sewing ring in order to obtain valve competence.

In this book, we discuss some of these important complex cardiac interventions using case studies. Imaging and interventional cardiologists work together to develop an inter-disciplinary team skill set that can then be adapted towards specific percutaneous procedures in order to ensure optimal patient outcome.

Chapter 1
Transcatheter Aortic Valve Implantation (TAVI)

Anitha Varghese, Neal Uren, and Peter F. Ludman

Transcatheter aortic valve implantation (TAVI) has evolved from novel technology to mainstream therapy in only a few years (Fig. 1.1). The first randomized trial was published in 2010 and 5 years on TAVI is available in more than 65 countries around the world, more than 200,000 valves have been implanted, and estimated global growth is projected to quadruple over the next 10 years. Valve sizing and positioning are crucial and require integration of information regarding type of valve being implanted, route of implantation, underlying anatomy of aortic valve and coronary artery origins, operator experience, and cardiac imaging techniques (Figs. 1.2 and 1.3). Procedures can be performed under a general anaesthetic with guidance from transoesophageal echocardiography (TOE) and 95 % of patients are extubated in the catheter laboratory. Transfemoral TAVI can also be performed using conscious sedation and local anaesthetic without TOE and in some countries this is the preferred technique. We present a case of TAVI performed in the United Kingdom (UK) in 2012 under general anaesthetic (available to view at www.mici.education).

Electronic supplementary material The online version of this chapter (doi:10.1007/978-1-4471-4981-1_1) contains supplementary material, which is available to authorized users.

A. Varghese, MD, MRCP (✉)
London, UK
e-mail: la@doctors.org.uk

N. Uren
Royal Infirmary of Edinburgh, Edinburgh, UK

P.F. Ludman, MD, FRCP
Queen Elizabeth Hospital, Birmingham, UK

A. Varghese et al. (eds.), *Cases in Structural Cardiac Intervention*,
DOI 10.1007/978-1-4471-4981-1_1

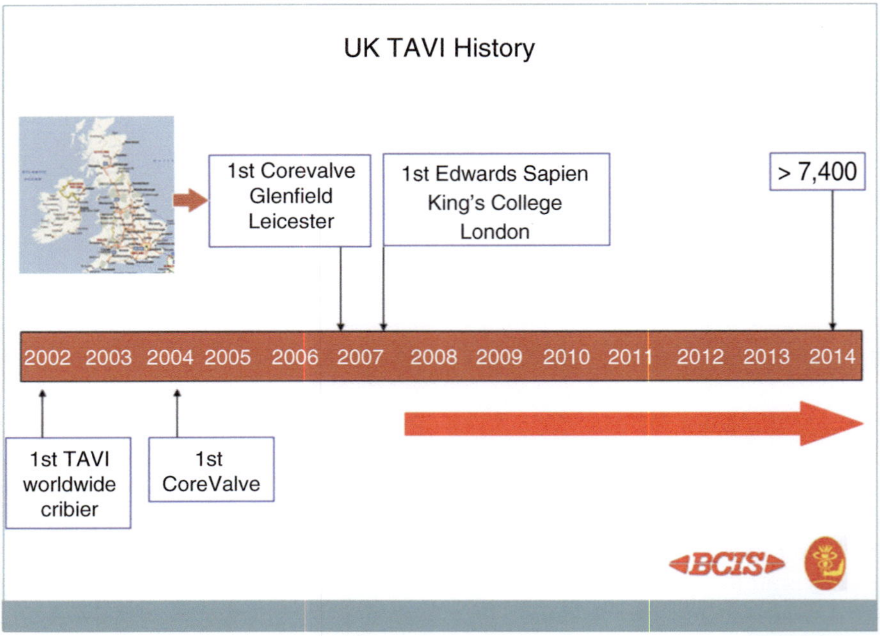

Fig. 1.1 Uptake of TAVI procedures in the United Kingdom

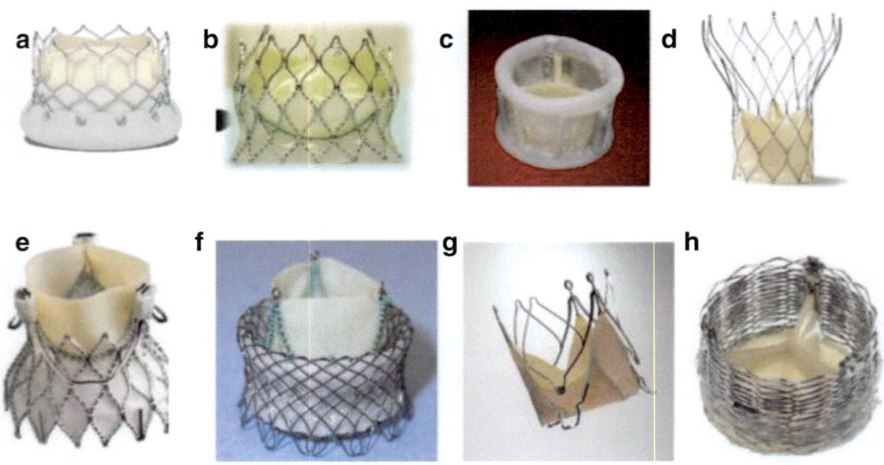

Fig. 1.2 Emerging TAVI Devices (**a**) SAPIEN 3 (Edwards Lifesciences, Irvine, California). (**b**) CENTERA (Edwards Lifesciences). (**c**) Direct Flow Medical (Direct Flow Medical, Santa Rosa, California). (**d**) Portico (St. Jude Medical, St. Paul, Minnesota). (**e**) Engager (Medtronic, Minneapolis, Minnesota). (**f**) Heart Leaflet Technologies (Heart Leaflet Technologies, Maple Grove, Minnesota). (**g**) JenaValve (JenaValve Technology, Munich, Germany). (**h**) Sadra Lotus Medical (Boston Scientific SciMed Inc., Maple Grove, Minnesota) (From *J Am Coll Cardiol*. 2013;61:1125–36)

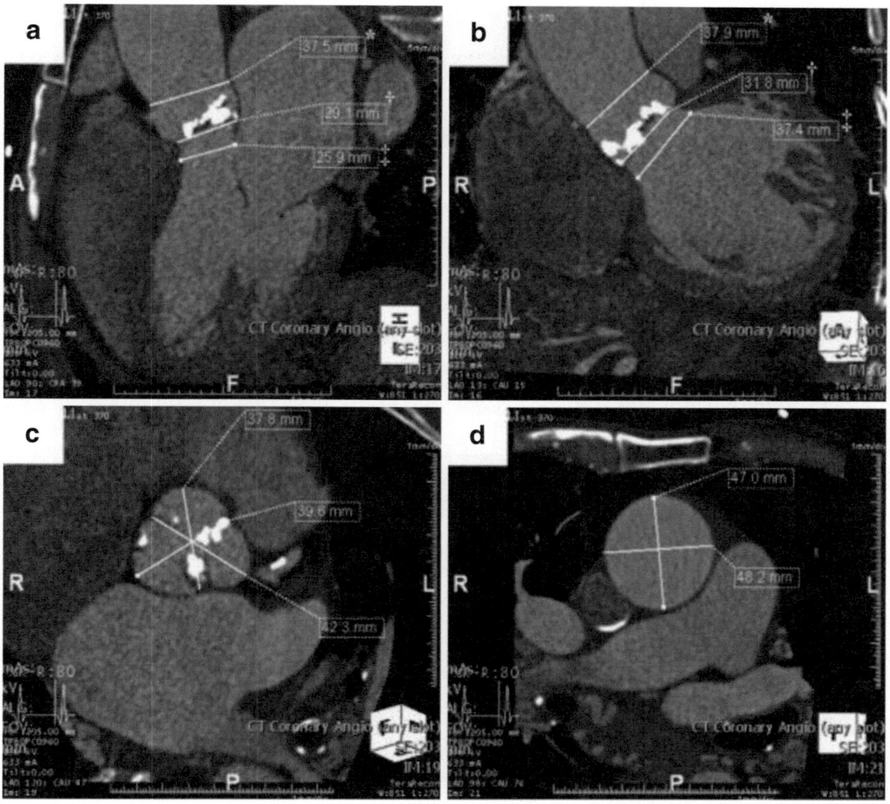

Fig. 1.3 Cardiac Computed Tomography of Aortic Root and Ascending Aorta demonstrating measurement of the sinotubular junction (*) and aortic annulus (†) in oblique-sagittal (**a**) and oblique-coronal (**b**) planes. Three-cusp commissure measurements (*arrows*) of the aortic sinuses were made from a short-axis image of the aortic root (**c**). The ascending aorta dimensions (*arrows*) were measured from a transaxial image at the level of the right pulmonary artery (**d**). (**a**, **b**) ‡denotes left ventricular out-flow tract measures (From *J Am Coll Cardiol*. 2011;58:2165–73)

Case Study

A 72 year old lady was referred for urgent aortic valve surgery (aortic valve replacement – AVR) for severe symptomatic calcific aortic stenosis in 2008. Additionally, she would require coronary artery revascularisation and tricuspid valve repair for concomitant coronary artery disease and severe tricuspid regurgitation.

Her predominant symptoms were exertional dyspnoea (New York Heart Association (NYHA) Class III), chest pain and dizziness. Past medical history included mechanical mitral valve replacement (MVR) in 2001, atrial fibrillation, peripheral vascular disease requiring intervention in 2000, and transsphenoidal hypophysectomy for acromegaly in 1996.

Transthoracic echocardiography (TTE) demonstrated an aortic valve area of 0.7 cm^2, mean aortic valve gradient 36 mmHg, and peak trans valvular velocity

4.1 m/s in the context of good left ventricular (LV) systolic function (Video 1.1; Fig. 1.4). TOE confirmed a stable bi-leaflet mechanical MVR with normal leaflet mobility (Video 1.2; Fig. 1.5). At both TTE and TOE, severe tricuspid regurgitation was measured and the right ventricle was noted to be dilated with preserved systolic function. Aortic root diameter was normal.

Exercise tolerance testing was indeterminate at a poor level of exercise. Cardiac catheterisation had shown stenoses in her right coronary artery (RCA) and left circumflex (LCx), but an unobstructed left main stem (LMS) and left anterior descending artery (LAD). Lung function tests and carotid Dopplers were normal, and the dental team had optimised dentition.

Following review by the cardiothoracic surgical team, the patient was considered too high risk for conventional AVR because of her previous mitral valve surgery, pulmonary hypertension and frailty. She was therefore discussed at a multidisciplinary

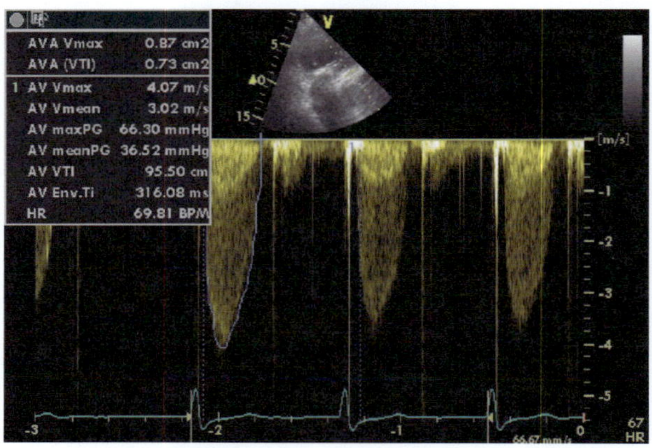

Fig. 1.4 Transthoracic echocardiography continuous wave Doppler confirming severe aortic stenosis

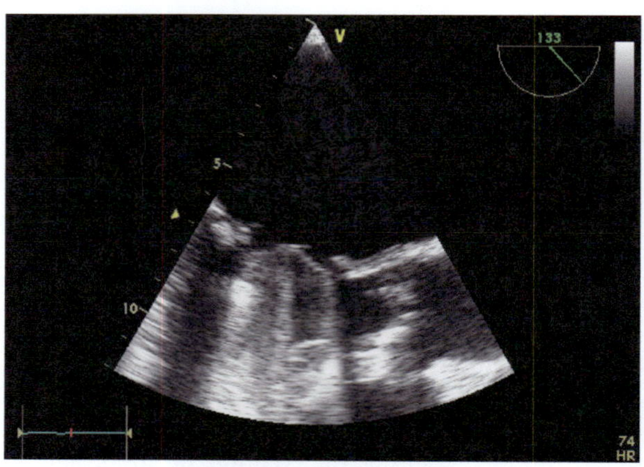

Fig. 1.5 Transoesophageal echocardiography demonstrating normal functioning of her bi-leaflet mechanical mitral valve replacement

team (MDT) meeting to assess suitability for TAVI. Despite ongoing symptoms, the patient was initially reluctant to undergo intervention and chose close clinic follow-up. Some 4 years later, in July 2012, after further symptomatic deterioration, she reconsidered this position and agreed to go ahead with treatment.

Repeat TTE showed that the valve had narrowed further with an area now measuring 0.6 cm^2. The patient was quoted the following risks for a TAVI procedure; 6–10 % mortality, 2–3 % risk of stroke, 5 % risk of requiring a permanent pacemaker, 5 % risk of access site complications, and a small risk of the need for renal replacement therapy.

This patient's investigations as work-up for TAVI included: updated biochemistry, left heart catheterization, TOE, spirometry, and carotid Dopplers; as well as right heart catheterization and computed tomography (CT) aortogram. Serum creatinine was 105 with an eGFR of 56 ml/min. The severity of her aortic stenosis had progressed so that at TOE, the aortic valve area was now 0.5 cm^2 with a peak velocity of 4.9 m/s and a mean gradient of 49 mmHg. Moderate central aortic regurgitation was seen and the aortic annulus dimension was quoted as 2.3 cm (Fig. 1.6). LV size and function remained normal. Left heart catheter showed mild distal attenuation of the LMS, moderate disease within the LAD and first diagonal, mild disease within a non-dominant LCx, and severe distal disease in the dominant RCA extending into the atrioventricular continuation (Video 1.3a, b). A decision was made not to perform percutaneous coronary revascularisation before TAVI, reserving this option only if she had on-going symptoms of chest pain after relief of her aortic stenosis. Right heart catheter study showed elevated pressures; pulmonary artery 45/15 mmHg with a mean 26 mmHg, pulmonary wedge mean pressure 17 mmHg with a v wave of 28 mmHg. CT aortogram showed moderate bilateral calcification of the iliofemoral vessels, the left external iliac with a diameter of 4.4 mm at its narrowest point and the right with a 4.7 mm diameter (Video 1.4a, b; Figs. 1.7a, b and 1.8). This degree of peripheral vascular disease precluded transfemoral access for TAVI (with the equipment available at that point in time). Based on these findings, the TAVI team

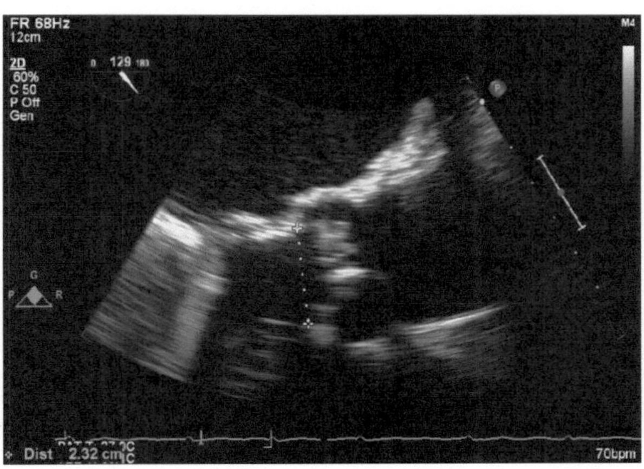

Fig. 1.6 Two-dimensional TOE measurement of aortic annulus diameter

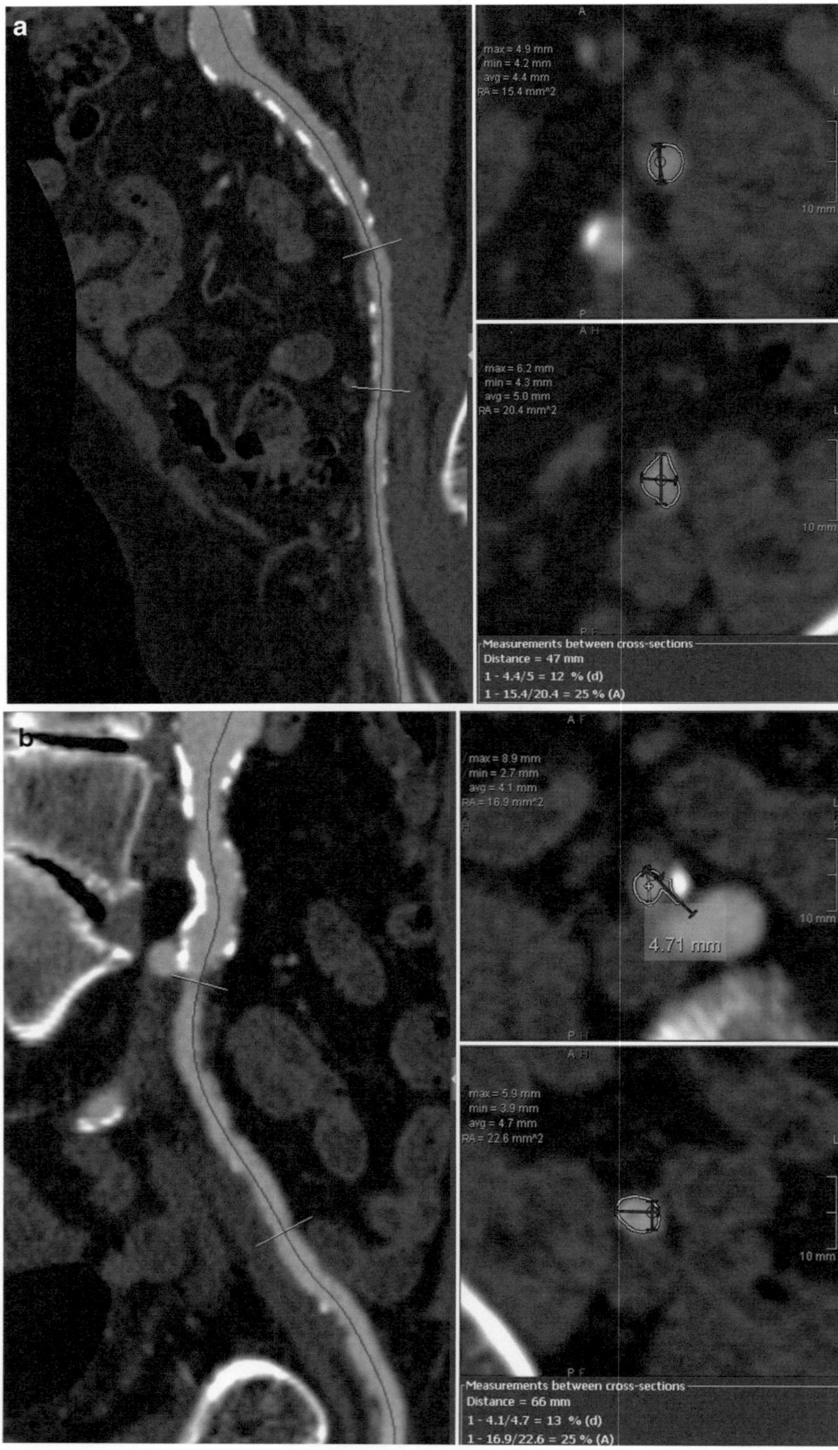

Fig. 1.7 Computed tomography multiplane reformat of iliofemoral system (**a** *left*, **b** *right*)

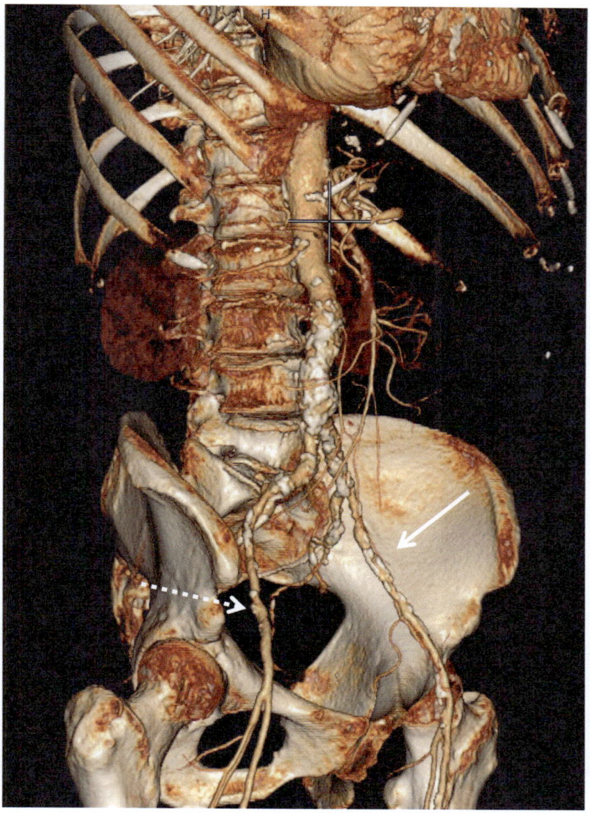

Fig. 1.8 Three-dimensional rendered computed tomogram of iliofemoral system (*left solid white arrow, right dashed white arrow*)

selected a direct aortic approach for implantation of a 26 mm Edwards Sapien XT valve. Logistic EuroSCORE was 35.

TAVI was performed in February 2013 under general anaesthetic. A right mini thoracotomy was performed for valve delivery. Access was also gained to the right femoral artery and vein for insertion of an aortic pigtail catheter and right ventricular pacing wire respectively. Repeat TOE measurements sized the aortic annulus at 25–26 mm (Video 1.5; Fig. 1.9). Balloon valvuloplasty with a 25 mm Crystal balloon and simultaneous aortography showed no paravalvular leak and so a 26 mm Sapien XT valve was positioned under fluoroscopic and TOE guidance with deployment during rapid burst pacing at 180 beats per minute. Post-procedure, no paravalvular leak was detected (Video 1.6). A single chest drain was placed in the right pleural space as the pericardium was open from previous thoracotomy.

The patient was transferred to the Intensive Care Unit (ITU) where heparin was given later the same evening to reduce the risk of thrombosis of her mechanical MVR. Unfortunately this induced bleeding requiring a further chest drain to be inserted in the right pleural space. Warfarin was re-established when the bleeding had stopped. A few days following hospital discharge, the patient was re-admitted

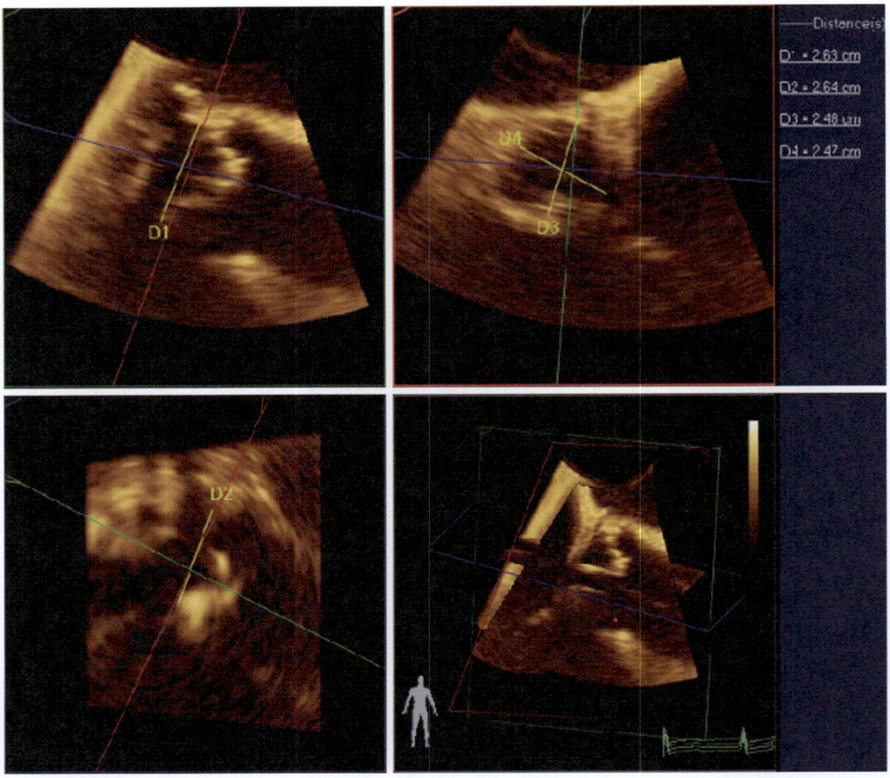

Fig. 1.9 Three-dimensional TOE measurements of aortic annulus size (Current annulus sizing is usually performed using cardiac computed tomography)

due to an embolic stroke causing right sided weakness and dysphasia. Head CT confirmed no haemorrhage. Aspirin was given but the combination of warfarin and an antiplatelet drug resulted in a gastrointestinal bleed and a haemorrhagic pleural effusion, which was drained. Post-operative hospital recovery was thus prolonged by a further 5 weeks.

At initial clinic review her dyspnoea was much improved. Speech remained impaired but no limb weakness was present. Surveillance TTE showed a stable well functioning TAVI prosthesis with minimal paravalvular leak (Video 1.7). At 2 year follow-up, she has no breathlessness or chest pain and mild residual expressive dysphasia.

Results of UK TAVI Programme 2007–2012

Between 2007 and 2012, 3980 TAVI implants were performed in the UK. Analysis of UK TAVI registry data has shown little change in characteristics of patients treated during that time. The only demographic shift was toward the treatment of patients with lower LV ejection fraction. In 2009, a UK TAVI Steering Group was formed and

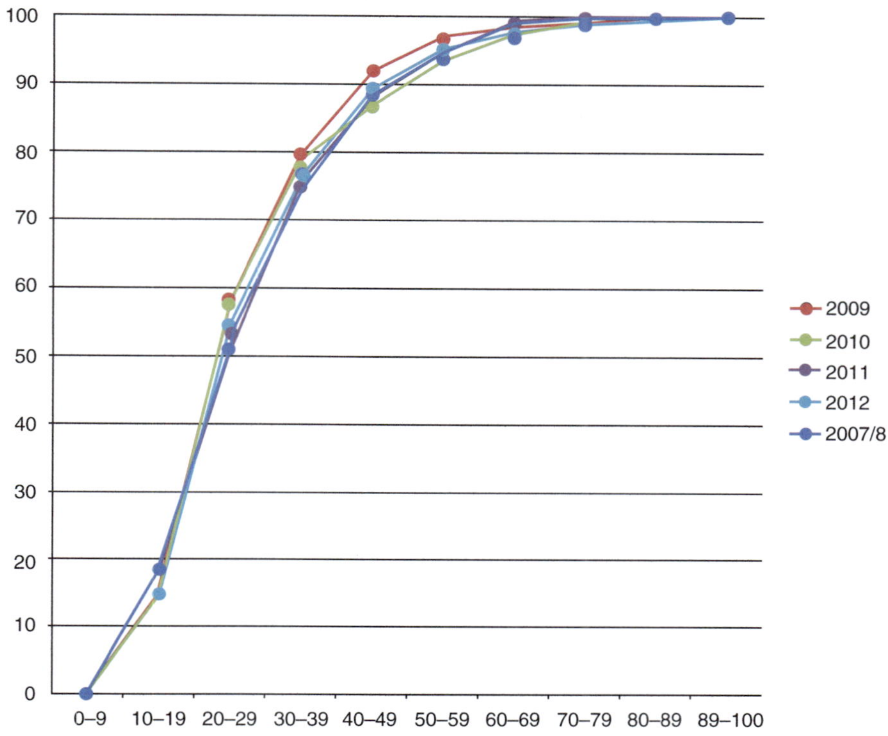

Fig. 1.10 Cumulative frequency plot of Logistic EuroSCORE for each of the annual cohorts of patients

their position statement mandated a MDT approach for the selection of patients, the requirement that TAVI is performed only in surgical centres, and the implication that funding would be restricted to the treatment of high-risk patients. 'High-risk' patients were defined using existing 'scoring' systems that aim to predict the risk of a patient not surviving surgery based on their pre-procedural characteristics and comorbidities. The cut-off for high-risk was suggested to be patients with a logistic EuroSCORE >20 and Society of Thoracic Surgeons score >10. Compliance to this guidance is likely responsible for lack of "EuroSCORE creep" (Fig. 1.10).

The only multivariate pre-procedural predictor of 30-day mortality was a Logistic EuroSCORE ≥40. There was no identified isolated pre-procedural multivariate predictor of 30-day outcome supporting the observation that TAVI is well tolerated in the elderly and consistent with lack of an accepted scoring system to predict early results. One-year survival was 81.7 %, falling to 37.3 % at 6 years with pre-procedural atrial fibrillation strongly associated with later mortality.

Patients who can be treated by a femoral route have a lower mortality than those for whom an alternative route is needed. Whether the direct aortic approach offers a lower operative risk than a transapical approach is not yet established. Theoretical benefits include less risk of apical rupture and delayed pseudoaneurysm formation, less interference with post-operative respiratory dynamics, and no risk to LV function caused by an apical purse-string suture. The use of the direct aortic approach has been increasing, but survival rates for this route versus transapical show no significant difference at 1–2 years.

There was a consistently low rate of peri-procedural stroke, but when this complication occurred it had the strongest independent association with a high early and late mortality (Fig. 1.11). Post-procedural aortic regurgitation was also a significant predictor of adverse outcome. Better outcomes were observed in patients with prior cardiac surgery and this remained a predictor of good outcome on multivariate analysis at 2 years.

By 2012, 30-day mortality, 1 year, and 2 year survival rates were improved compared to 2007 UK TAVI registry results.

Future of TAVI

This technology has seen a rapid worldwide acceptance and lower risk patient groups are likely to undergo TAVI in the future. Trial data and patient choice will be crucial factors in this fundamental change in the treatment of aortic stenosis. Recent studies of patient in the 'intermediate' risk group suggest that TAVI has similar

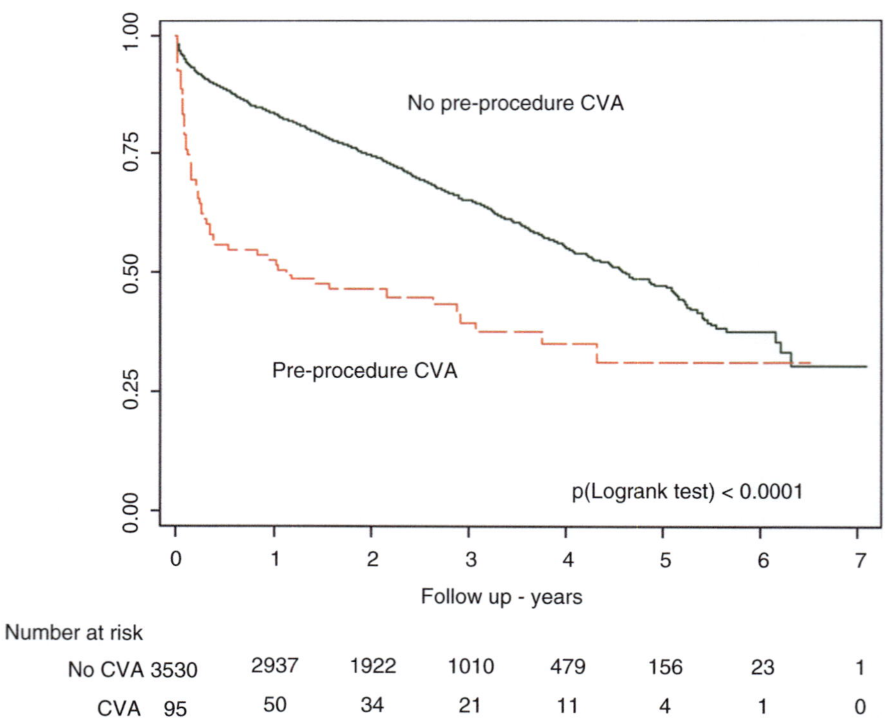

Fig. 1.11 Kaplan–Meier survival curves from UK TAVI Registry showing survival according to peri-procedural cerebrovascular accident (CVA)

outcomes to surgery. Success with deployment in the aortic position has led to operators considering this procedure in critically ill patients with valve disease at other sites, and TAVI to treat other valves has already begun.

Recommended Reading

1. Nishimura RA, Otto CM, Bonow RO et al. 2014 AHA/ACC Guideline for the management of patients with valvular heart disease. Circulation. 2014;129:e521–e623.
2. Adams DH, Popma JJ, Reardon MJ et al. Transcatheter aortic-valve replacement with a self-expanding prosthesis-CoreValve US Pivotal high-risk study. N Engl J Med. 2014;370:1790–8.
3. Leon M, Smith CR, Mack MJ et al. Transcatheter or surgical aortic-valve replacement in intermediate-risk patients - PARTNER 2. N Engl J Med. 2016;374:1609–20.
4. Leon MB, Smith CR, Mack M et al. Transcatheter aortic-valve implantation for aortic stenosis in patients who cannot undergo surgery - PARTNER Trial. N Engl J Med. 2010;363:1597–607.

Chapter 2
Left Atrial Appendage Closure (LAAC)

Anitha Varghese, Patrick Calvert, and Peter F. Ludman

Atrial fibrillation (AF) affects approximately 15 million patients worldwide and carries an increased risk of stroke. It is estimated that 90 % of stroke comes from embolism of left atrial appendage (LAA) thrombus in non-valvular AF. The concept of mechanical occlusion of the LAA to reduce stroke risk has been refined over the years since it was first done surgically. Although anticoagulants such as warfarin are used to reduce stroke risk in AF and the new oral anticoagulants (novel oral anticoagulants or NOACs) are of benefit in non-valvular AF, bleeding remains a continuous risk in a significant minority of patients.

From these observations the concept of an interventional approach to permanent occlusion of the LAA gained traction with the publication of the PROTECT AF (The *Watchman™* Left Atrial Appendage Closure (LAAC) Device for Embolic PROTECTion in Patients with Atrial Fibrillation) and PREVAIL (Prospective Randomized Evaluation of the *Watchman™* LAA Closure Device in Patients with Atrial Fibrillation Versus Long Term Warfarin Therapy) trials leading to CE mark approval of the *Watchman™* LAAC device in Europe in 2005, with alternative devices also now available such as the *Amplatzer™ Amulet™* which allows treatment of a wider range of appendage anatomies (Fig. 2.1). Indications for device

Electronic supplementary material The online version of this chapter (doi:10.1007/978-1-4471-4981-1_2) contains supplementary material, which is available to authorized users.

A. Varghese, MD, MRCP
London, UK
e-mail: la@doctors.org.uk

P. Calvert, PhD, MRCP (✉)
Papworth Hospital NHS Foundation Trust, Papworth Everard, Cambridge, UK
e-mail: paddy@doctors.org.uk

P.F. Ludman, FD, FRCP
Queen Elizabeth Hospital, Birmingham, UK

A. Varghese et al. (eds.), *Cases in Structural Cardiac Intervention*,
DOI 10.1007/978-1-4471-4981-1_2

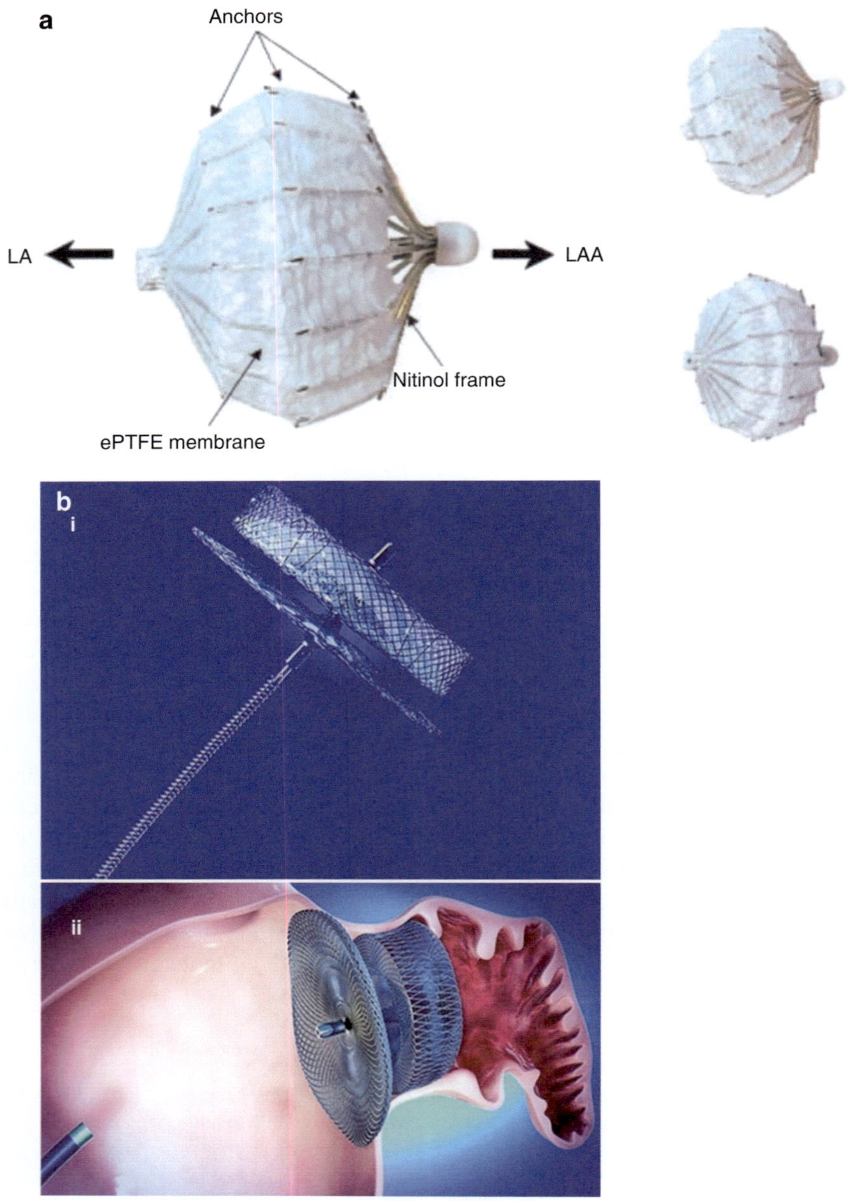

Fig. 2.1 Shown are several LAAC devices. (**a**) Percutaneous left atrial appendage transcatheter occlusion device (PLAATO). This was the first device available for percutaneous appendage closure and is no longer in use. (**b**) i) and ii) Amplatzer Cardiac Plug (ACP) which is in widespread use, to possibly be superseded by the next generation of device called the Amplatzer Amulet (St. Jude Medical, Inc., Plymouth, MN). (**c**) Amplatzer amulet LAA occluder device. This was developed for easier delivery and better coverage than the ACP and ss designed with a longer lobe and waist. (**d**) i) and ii) The Watchman device (Boston Scientific Corp., Natick, MA). The device comes in 5 different sizes: 21, 24, 27, 30, and 33 mm. (**e**) The wavecrest device (Coherex Medical, Inc., Salt Lake City, UT). This is composed of a nitinol frame covered by a non-thrombogenic expanded polytetrafluoroethylene membrane and is available in 3 sizes: 22, 27 or 32 mm

Fig. 2.1 (continued)

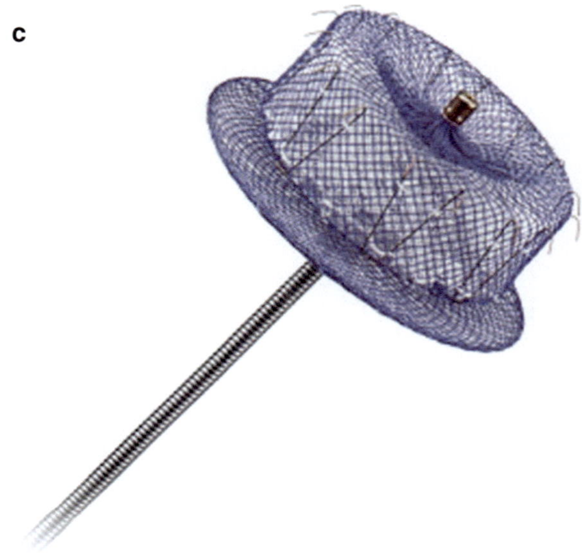

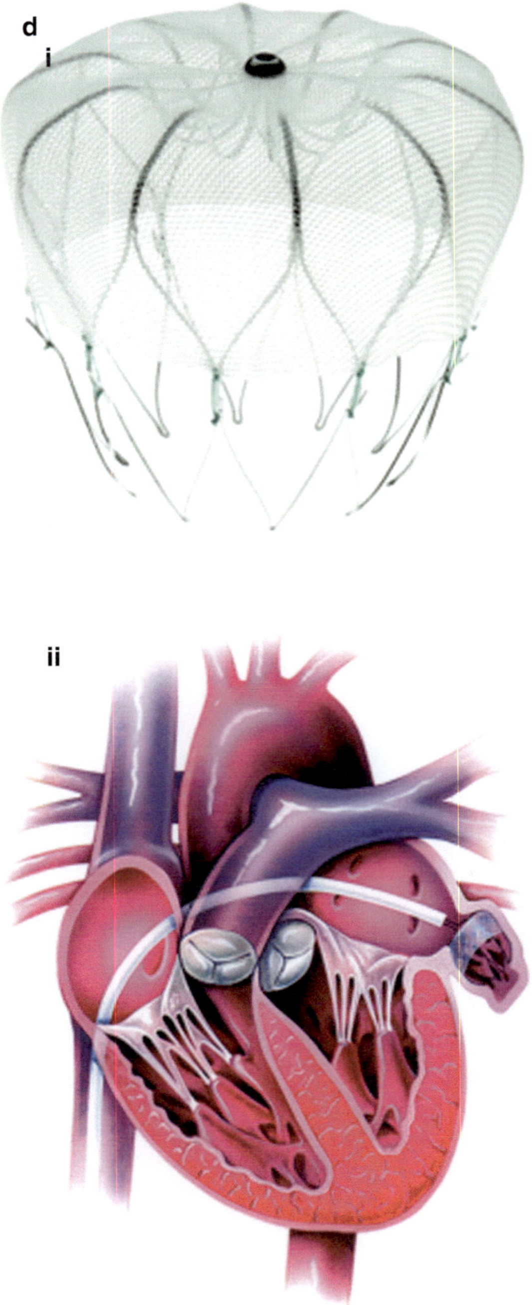

Fig. 2.1 (continued)

Fig. 2.1 (continued)

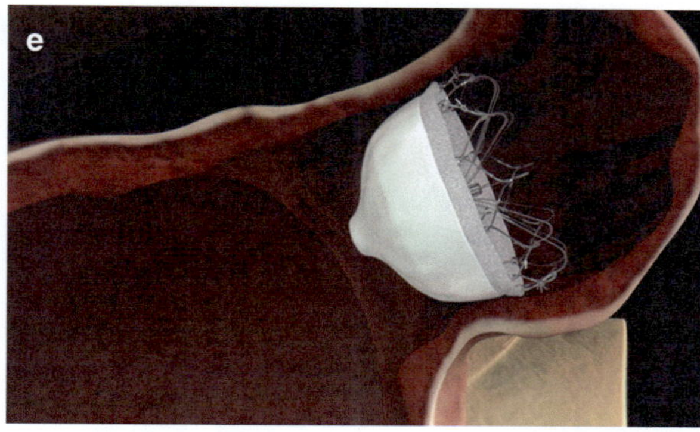

implantation include patients with non-valvular AF in whom warfarin is a contraindication or patients with AF who have cerebrovascular events despite optimal anticoagulation.

Case Study

A 73 year old man was transferred as an emergency in November 2014 to the neurosurgical team for left burr-hole evacuation of left subacute subdural haematoma on a background of warfarin anticoagulation for non-valvular AF (Fig. 2.2a). Presenting symptoms were right-sided weakness and reduced Glasgow Coma Scale (GCS 13 – Eye opening 3 Verbal response 4 Motor response 6). Past medical history included AF and ischaemic stroke, hypertension, and non-insulin-dependent diabetes mellitus. CHA_2DS_2-VASc risk score was calculated as 5, but rising to 6 in 2 years' time (Table 2.1).

Post-operatively, the cardiology team were consulted by the neurosurgeons. Due to the high risk of recurrent ischaemic stroke in association with satisfactory resolution of the left subdural haematoma, re-initiation of warfarin after 6 weeks was advised with simultaneous referral for placement of a LAAC device. The patient was discharged with GCS 15 and a Falls Assessment indicating that he remained at risk of falls.

At outpatient neurosurgical review in February 2015 he complained of a deterioration in balance, gait, and memory for the preceding few weeks. The international normalised ratio (INR) was therapeutic at 2.8. Urgent head computed tomography (CT) demonstrated that he had now developed a chronic subdural haematoma on the right side which was drained the next day. The patient again made a good recovery and was discharged 3 days following this second burr-hole operation. Warfarin was now permanently discontinued.

At outpatient cardiology review in March 2015 he was advised that risk of thromboembolic events was around 10 % per annum without anticoagulation and restarting warfarin would risk a further intracranial haemorrhage. LAAC was described and discussed, and initial investigations (transoesophageal echocardiogram (TOE) and

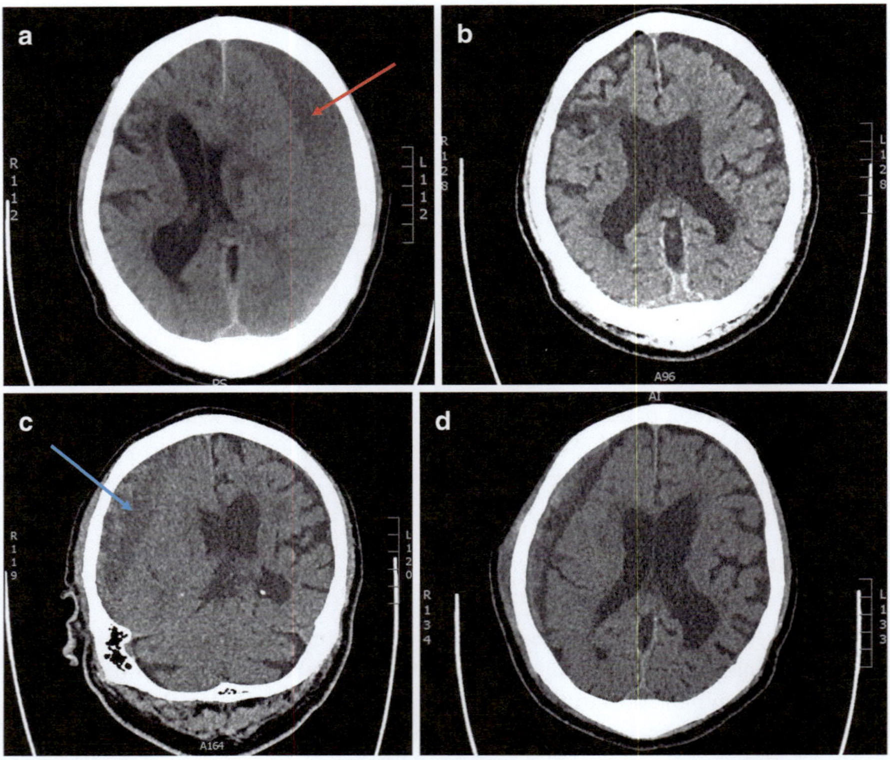

Fig. 2.2 A series of computed tomographic scans of the patent's head. (**a**) Large left subacute subdural haematoma (*red arrow*) with mass effect and midline shift. (**b**) Following surgical evacuation of the haematoma there is marked improvement in mass effect. There remains bilateral convexity with subdural fluid collections, larger on the left. There is minor distortion of the midline but no significant midline shift. Scattered locules of postoperative pneumocephalus are present. No hydrocephalus. There is also an old right frontal and insular middle cerebral artery territory infarct, and advanced small vessel ischaemia. (**c**) Large right chronic subdural haematoma (*blue arrow*). There is a mixed density but mainly intermediate density collection overlying the right cerebral hemisphere causing mass effect and midline shift toward the left, with partial effacement of the left lateral ventricle. Strands of high density are present within this extraaxial collection, suggesting that there is some organisation within the haematoma and that it is not acute. (**d**) Following surgical evacuation of the right-sided haematoma there is marked improvement in mass effect. There is less midline shift and less effacement of the convexity sulci. No significant interval change to the subdural overlying the left frontal convexity

cardiac CT) were requested pending multi-disciplinary team review regarding suitability. Pre-procedural TOE performed in April 2015 showed a severely dilated left atrium (6.9 cm), no thrombus within the LAA in the presence of reduced emptying velocity (0.2 m/s), and a windsock appendage morphology with a shallow laterally directed additional lobe present proximally (Video 2.1). The LAA ostium diameter was measured as 28 mm on three-dimensional (3D) TOE, with a diameter 1 cm within the appendage of 16 mm (Fig. 2.3). Percutaneous LAAC was performed in June 2015 under general anaesthetic via the right femoral vein with TOE guidance.

Table 2.1 CHA_2DS_2-VASc risk score

	Condition	Points
C	Congestive heart failure (or Left ventricular systolic dysfunction)	1
H	Hypertension: blood pressure consistently above 140/90 mmHg (or treated hypertension on medication)	1
A_2	Age ≥75 years	2
D	Diabetes Mellitus	1
S_2	Prior Stroke or TIA or thromboembolism	2
V	Vascular disease (e.g., peripheral artery disease, myocardial infarction, aortic plaque)	1
A	Age 65–74 years	1
Sc	Sex category (i.e., female sex)	1

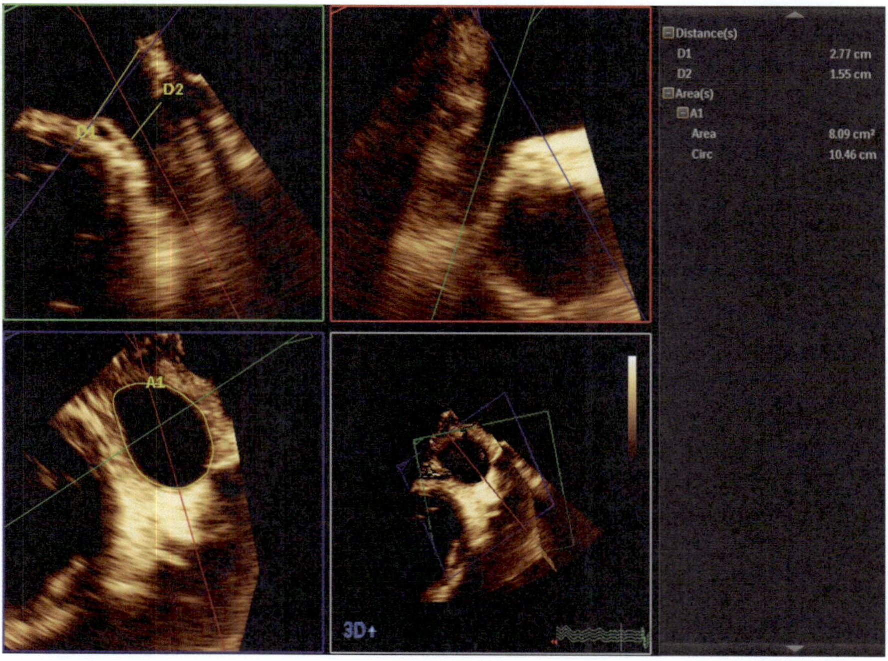

Fig. 2.3 Measurements of LAA anatomy from pre-procedural 3D TOE. TOE showed a measurement of 16 mm (D2) for the LAA diameter along a line that connects the position of the left circumflex coronary artery to a point 2 cm from the tip of the left upper pulmonary vein limbus, also known as the warfarin ridge. These measurements serve as a guide before the procedure and need to be repeated during the procedure once the left atrial pressure is confirmed to be above 10 mmHg

LAA morphology was confirmed angiographically (Video 2.2). The size of the appendage was re-assessed once it was confirmed that the left atrial pressure was above 10 mmHg, and a 27 mm *Watchman*^{TM} device was selected (Fig. 2.4a, b). At first attempted device deployment, the position was too distal necessitating partial recapture (this device cannot be reused following full recapture). The second deployment

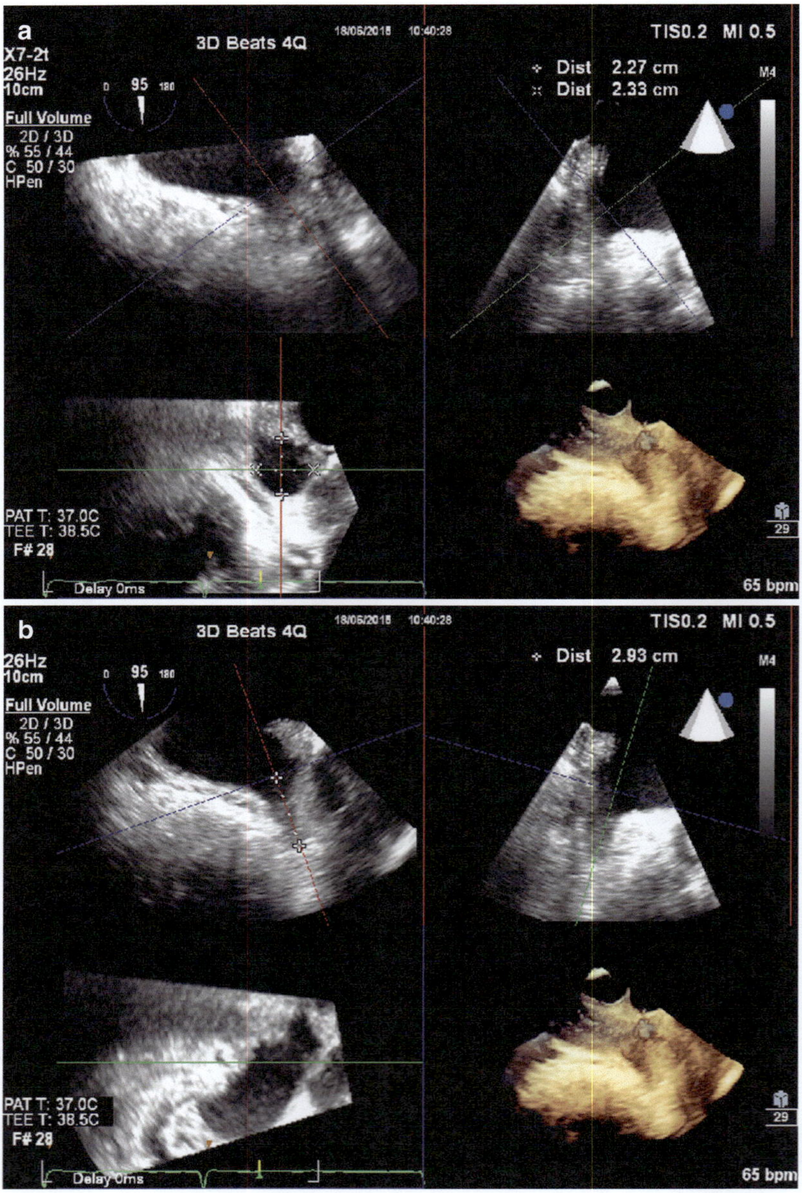

Fig. 2.4 3D TOE LAA assessment during procedure. Thrombus remained absent on a background of an INR $\geq$ 1.5, and following assessment of left atrial pressure (>10 mmHg) device sizing was performed. The LAA was measured in at least 4 TOE views: initially at 0° along a line from the left coronary artery to a point 2 cm from the warfarin ridge. Then measurements are made at 45, 90, and 135° from the top of the mitral valve annulus to a point 2 cm from the tip of the left upper pulmonary vein limbus. LAA ostium size should be >17 mm or <31 mm to accommodate available *Watchman*™ device sizes. (**a**) TOE measurements during the procedure demonstrated a suitable LAA ostial size of 23 mm, indicating the requirement for deployment of a 27 mm device according to the manufacturer's guidance on instructions for use. (**b**) LAA length should be $\geq$ the ostial diameter, as in this case

was more proximal and covered both lobes of the LAA (Video 2.3a, b; Fig. 2.5). The device was released (Video 2.4).

Device stability was confirmed with gentle retraction of the delivery mechanism and peri-procedural TOE showed appropriate compression of the device, measuring 24 mm (lying within the required 80–92 % of initial device size) with no colour leak (Video 2.5; Fig. 2.6). Post-procedural transthoracic echocardiogram demonstrated no significant pericardial effusion. The patient was discharged the next day on dual antiplatelet therapy with clopidogrel 75 mg and aspirin 75 mg for 6 weeks. Follow-up TOE from August 2015 confirmed a well seated device within the LAA, no throm-

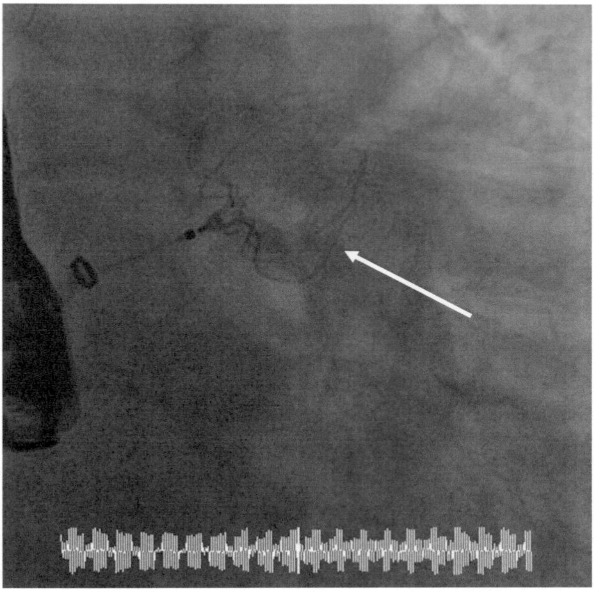

Fig. 2.5 Angiographic image of optimal *Watchman*™ device position in the LAA (*white arrow*)

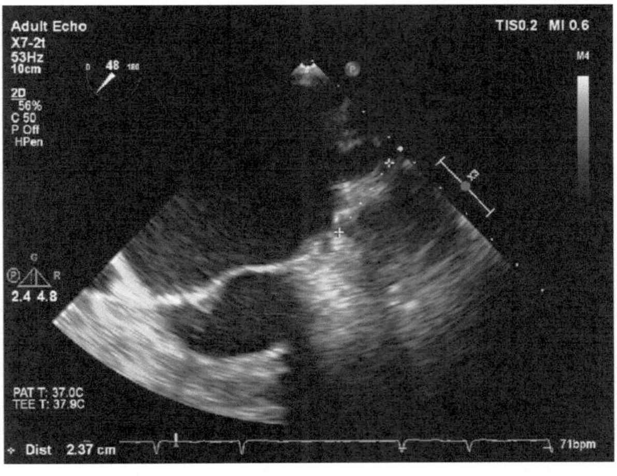

Fig. 2.6 Post-procedural assessment of satisfactory device compression. Device diameter measures 24 mm and therefore is within 80–92 % of initial device diameter

bus, and no significant leak around the implant. Clopidogrel was therefore discontinued, leaving aspirin monotherapy for the next 6 months.

Evidence Base for Left Atrial Appendage Closure

The PROTECT AF trial was designed to evaluate whether systemic anticoagulation with warfarin could be replaced by closure of the LAA with the percutaneously deployed *Watchman™* filter device. The device made of self-expanding nitinol with a polyethylene terephthalate cap is implanted within the LAA via a transseptal approach and anchored in place through fixation hooks. The PROTECT AF investigators hypothesized that the LAAC device would prove non-inferior to warfarin for the composite primary efficacy end point of stroke, systemic embolism, and cardiovascular death. Over 18 months follow-up in 707 patients with non-valvular AF randomised 2:1 to the *Watchman™* device there was a 38 % reduction in the composite primary endpoint. A total of 87 % of patients were able to discontinue warfarin after 45 days of deployment, and in this subgroup the reduction in the primary endpoint was 60 %. With regard to secondary endpoints of cardiovascular and all-cause mortality, there were significant reductions of 60 % and 36 % respectively. Study protocol required continuation of warfarin for at least 45 days after LAAC and TOE was repeated at 45 days, 6 months, and 1 year post implant. If imaging was satisfactory at the day 45 TOE assessment, warfarin was replaced with clopidogrel and aspirin dual antiplatelet treatment until 6 months, after which aspirin monotherapy could be continued lifelong.

After 1588 patient-years of follow-up (mean 2.3 ± 1.1 years), primary efficacy event rates were 3.0 and 4.3 % (percent per 100 patient-years) in the *Watchman™* and warfarin groups respectively (relative risk, 0.71; 95 % confidence interval, 0.44–1.30 % per year), which fulfills criteria of non-inferiority. However, the LAAC arm did sustain an increased number of procedure-related safety events, mainly pericardial tamponade and procedure-related stroke perhaps related to the early learning curve of many enrolling centres. After successful deployment, the local therapy of LAAC proved superior to well-controlled systemic anticoagulation, and this is particularly true when the functional impact of major adverse clinical events was considered.

At 2621 patient-years of follow-up (mean 3.8 ± 1.7 years) in patients with non-valvular AF, device closure met criteria for both non-inferiority and superiority, compared with warfarin, for the prevention of the combined outcome of stroke, systemic embolism, and cardiovascular death, as well as superiority for cardiovascular and all-cause mortality.

The PREVAIL trial assessed the safety and efficacy of the *Watchman™* device over 18 months. Patients with non-valvular AF who had a CHADS2 score ≥ 2 or 1 and another risk factor were enrolled and randomized in a 2:1 ratio as follows: LAAC and subsequent discontinuation of warfarin (intervention group, n = 269) versus chronic warfarin therapy (control group, n = 138). After successful implantation, 92.2, 98.3, and 99.3 % of patients were able to discontinue warfarin after

45 days, 6 months, and 12 months respectively. Two efficacy and one safety co-primary endpoints were evaluated between intervention and control groups. The first co-primary efficacy endpoint was a composite of rate of stroke, systemic embolism, and cardiovascular/unexplained death. The second co-primary efficacy endpoint was rate of stroke or systemic embolism >7 days' post randomization. Only this second efficacy endpoint achieved non-inferiority for the device closure cohort. Early safety events occurred in 2.2 % of the *Watchman™* arm. Using a more inclusive definition of adverse effects, procedure–related event rates were 4.2 % in PREVAIL versus 8.7 % in PROTECT AF ($p = 0.004$). Pericardial effusions requiring surgical repair decreased from 1.6 % to 0.4 % ($p = 0.027$), and those requiring pericardiocentesis decreased from 2.9 % to 1.5 % ($p = 0.36$), although the number of events was small.

Future of LAAC

LAAC will have an expanding role as second-line therapy in AF as more tertiary centres become experienced in its use. The individual clinical setting and the patient's informed decision regarding lifelong anticoagulation will also be key determinants on the rate of uptake of this important technology.

Recommended Reading

1. Holmes Jr DR, Kar S, Price MJ et al. Prospective randomized evaluation of the *Watchman™* left atrial appendage closure device in patients with atrial fibrillation versus long-term warfarin therapy: the PREVAIL trial. J Am Coll Cardiol. 2014;64:1–12.
2. Holmes DR, Reddy VY, Turi ZG et al. Percutaneous closure of the left atrial appendage versus warfarin therapy for prevention of stroke in patients with atrial fibrillation: a randomised non-inferiority trial. Lancet. 2009;374:534–42.
3. Reddy VY, Doshi SK, Sievert H et al. Percutaneous left atrial appendage closure for stroke prophylaxis in patients with atrial fibrillation: 2.3-year follow-up of the PROTECT AF (*Watchman™* left atrial appendage system for embolic protection in patients with atrial fibrillation) trial. Circulation. 2013;127:720–9.
4. Reddy VY, Sievert H, Halperin J et al. Percutaneous left atrial appendage closure vs warfarin for atrial fibrillation: a randomized clinical trial. JAMA. 2014;312:1988–98.

Chapter 3
Percutaneous Coronary Intervention of Chronic Total Occlusion (CTO)

Anitha Varghese and Peter F. Ludman

For patients with limiting angina in spite of medical therapy coronary revascularisation either by coronary artery bypass grafting (CABG) or percutaneous coronary intervention (PCI) is extremely efficacious for symptom relief. Whether to treat using the surgical option or by PCI is decided by several factors which impact on the relative efficacy of each technique. These include a patient's presenting coronary syndrome, their co-morbidities and their coronary anatomy. Coronary artery stenoses usually pose little challenge to current percutaneous techniques. During PCI, the aim is to cross the diseased segment of vessel with a fine guidewire (0.014″ in diameter), dilate the narrowed lumen and implant a stent to scaffold the vessel walls open. The wire is steered by rotating and advancing its curved tip through the vessel lumen until it sits in a distal position and can provide a rail to introduce subsequent equipment such as angioplasty balloons and stents. Difficulties are encountered when treating heavily calcified vessels and where atheroma sits at bifurcations or trifurcations, but arguably the most challenging subset of lesion to treat by PCI are those which are chronically occluded.

A chronic total occlusion (CTO) is characterised by heavy atherosclerotic plaque burden within the coronary artery resulting in complete obstruction of the vessel. The definition of a CTO is an obstruction that has been present for at least 3 months, but duration of occlusion can be hard to determine on clinical grounds. During PCI of a CTO, rather than the guidewire following within the lumen of the vessel the operator re-canalises the vessel by penetrating the fibrocalcific material of the CTO using the wire before re-entering the distal vessel lumen of the coronary artery

---

Electronic supplementary material The online version of this chapter (doi:10.1007/978-1-4471-4981-1_3) contains supplementary material, which is available to authorized users.

A. Varghese, MD, MRCP (✉)
London, UK
e-mail: la@doctors.org.uk

P.F. Ludman, MA, MD, FRCP
Queen Elizabeth Hospital, Birmingham, UK

A. Varghese et al. (eds.), *Cases in Structural Cardiac Intervention*,
DOI 10.1007/978-1-4471-4981-1_3

(available to view at www.mici.education). An occlusion can be crossed anterogradely or retrogradely, and the guidewire can cross either through the atheromatous plaque or outside the plaque in the arterial wall (Fig. 3.1a, b).

Increasingly sophisticated guidewires have been developed for arterial tissue penetration and easier steering through lesions (Table 3.1). If an occlusion cannot be

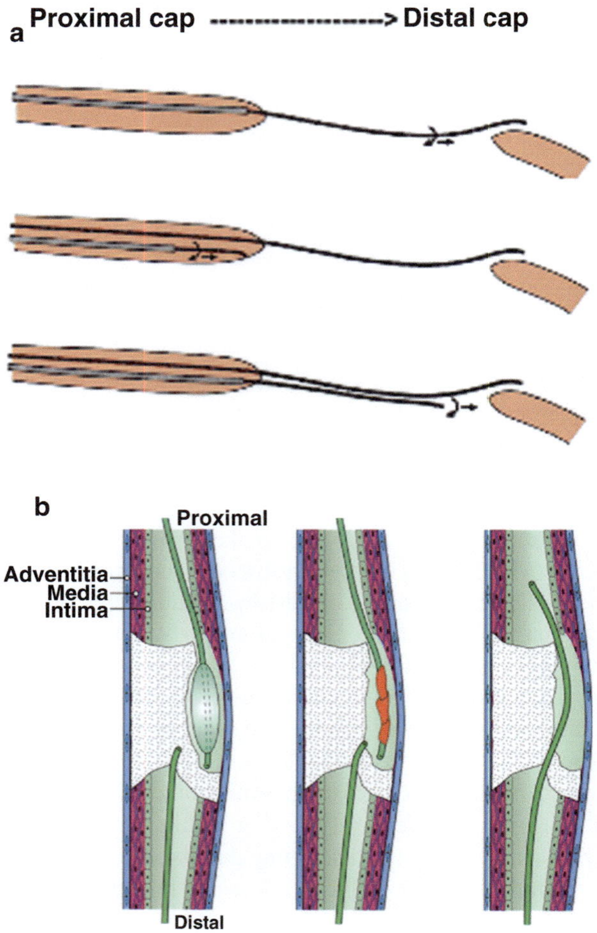

Fig. 3.1 An example of one antegrade and retrograde technique for crossing a CTO. (**a**) The antegrade approach requires defined proximal cap anatomy ideally with a tapered stump or defined entry point. In *parallel wiring*, a first wire is passed into the subintimal space and left in position to seal that tract and act as a marker, while avoiding the cap of the distal true lumen. A second penetrating wire is then introduced via a microcatheter to attempt redirection into the true lumen. (**b**) The retrograde approach is usually reserved as a second line strategy for failed intimal antegrade crossing but suggested as a first line where the proximal stump is ambiguous. In the reverse controlled anterograde and retrograde tracking and dissection (reverse CART) technique a balloon is inflated over the antegrade wire within the subintimal (subluminal) space that is connected proximally to the true lumen. The retrograde wire is advanced toward the newly created space

Table 3.1 An overview of currently available wires used in CTO

Wire	Manufacturer	Design/lengths	Coating	Tip load (g)	Penetration force kg/in.^{2}
Fielder FC	Asahi	Non-tapered tip. 0.014 in., 180 and 300 cm lengths.	Hydrophilic, polymer jacket	0.8	N/A
Fielder XT	Asahi	Tapered tip 0.009 in. Shaft 0.014 in., 180 and 300 cm lengths	Hydrophilic, polymer jacket	0.8	N/A
Fielder XT – A (A for antegrade)	Asahi	Tapered tip 0.009 in. Shaft 0.014 in., 180 and 300 cm lengths	Hydrophilic, polymer jacket	1.0	N/A
Fielder XT – R (R for retrograde collateral cross)	Asahi	Tapered tip 0.009 in. Shaft 0.014 in., 180 and 300 cm lengths	Hydrophilic, polymer jacket	0.6	N/A
Pilot 50	Abbott	Non-tapered tip. 0.014 in., 190 and 300 cm lengths	Hydrophilic, polymer jacket	1.5	N/A
Sion For retrograde collateral cross	Asahi	Non-Tapered tip. 0.014 in., 180 and 300 cm lengths	Hydrophilic, non-jacketed over spring coil and tip.	0.7	N/A
Sion blue Workhorse wire for procedure completion	Asahi	Non-Tapered tip. 0.014 in., 180 and 300 cm lengths	Hydrophilic, non-jacketed over spring coil. Hydrophobic tip.	0.5	N/A
Gaia first	Asahi	Tapered tip 0.010 in. Shaft 0.014 in., 190 cm	Hydrophilic, non-jacketed. Tip hydrophilic	1.5	Penetration efficiency rather than power. On par with miracle 6
Gaia second	Asahi	Tapered tip 0.011 in. Shaft 0.014 in., 190 cm	Hydrophilic, non-jacketed. Tip hydrophilic	3.5	Penetration efficiency rather than power. On par with miracle 12

(continued)

Table 3.1 (continued)

Wire	Manufacturer	Design/lengths	Coating	Tip load (g)	Penetration force kg/in.^{2}
Gaia third	Asahi	Tapered tip 0.011 in. Shaft 0.014 in., 190 cm	Hydrophilic, non-jacketed. Tip hydrophilic	4.5	Penetration efficiency rather than power. On par with Conquest Pro 12
Miracle 3/ MIRACLEbros 3	Asahi	Non-tapered tip. 0.014 in., 180 cm length	Hydrophobic (silicone)	3.0	20
Miracle 4.5/ MIRACLEbros 4.5	Asahi	Non-tapered tip. 0.014 in., 180 cm length	Hydrophobic (silicone)	4.5	30
Miracle 6/ MIRACLEbros 6	Asahi	Non-tapered tip. 0.014 in., 180 cm length	Hydrophobic (silicone)	6.0	39
Miracle 12/ MIRACLEbros 12	Asahi	Non-tapered tip. 0.014 in., 180 cm length	Hydrophobic (silicone)	12.0	78
Ultimate Bros 3	Asahi	Non-tapered tip. 0.014 in., 180 and 300 cm lengths	Hydrophilic, non-jacketed	3	20
Pilot 150	Abbott	Non-tapered tip. 0.014 in., 190 and 300 cm length	Hydrophilic, polymer jacketed	2.7	N/A
Pilot 200	Abbott	Non-tapered tip. 0.014 in., 190 and 300 cm length	Hydrophilic, polymer jacketed	4.1	N/A
Conquest/ Confianza	Asahi	Tapered tip 0.009 in. Shaft 0.014 in. 180 cm length. Spring coil length 20 cm	Hydrophobic (silicone)	9.0	142
Conquest Pro/ Confianza Pro	Asahi	Tapered tip 0.009 in. Shaft 0.014 in., 180 cm length. Spring coil length 20 cm	Hydrophilic non-jacketed over spring coil. Hydrophobic tip and shaft	9.0	142

Table 3.1 (continued)

Wire	Manufacturer	Design/lengths	Coating	Tip load (g)	Penetration force kg/in.^{2}
Conquest Pro 12/ Confianza Pro 12	Asahi	Tapered tip 0.009 in. Shaft 0.014 in., 180 cm length. Spring coil length 20 cm	Hydrophilic non-jacketed over spring coil. Hydrophobic tip and shaft	12.0	189
Conquest Pro 8–20/Confianza Pro 8–20	Asahi	Tapered tip 0.009 in. Shaft 0.014 in., 180 cm length. Spring coil length 17 cm	Hydrophilic non-jacketed over spring coil. Hydrophobic tip and shaft	20.0	315
High torque CROSS IT 100 XT	Abbott	Tapered tip 0.010 in. Shaft 0.014 in. 190 and 300 cm length.	Hydrophilic including tip, non-jacketed	1.7	22
High torque CROSS IT 200 XT	Abbott	Tapered tip 0.010 in. Shaft 0.014 in. 190 and 300 cm length.	Hydrophilic including tip, non-jacketed	4.7	60
High torque CROSS IT 300 XT	Abbott	Tapered tip 0.010 in. Shaft 0.014 in. 190 and 300 cm length.	Hydrophilic including tip, non-jacketed	6.2	79
High torque CROSS IT 400 XT	Abbott	Tapered tip 0.010 in. Shaft 0.014 in. 190 and 300 cm length.	Hydrophilic including tip, non-jacketed	8.7	110
High torque Progress 40	Abbott	Non-Tapered tip 0.014 in. 190 and 300 cm length.	Hydrophilic, non-jacketed.	4.8	30
High torque Progress 80	Abbott	Non-Tapered tip 0.014 in. 190 and 300 cm length.	Hydrophilic, non-jacketed.	9.7	63
High torque Progress 120	Abbott	Non-Tapered tip 0.014 in. 190 and 300 cm length.	Hydrophilic, non-jacketed.	13.9	90

(continued)

Table 3.1 (continued)

Wire	Manufacturer	Design/lengths	Coating	Tip load (g)	Penetration force kg/in.^{2}
High torque Progress 140T	Abbott	Tapered tip 0.0105 in. Shaft 0.014 in. 190 and 300 cm length.	Hydrophilic, non-jacketed.	12.5	144
High torque Progress 200T	Abbott	Tapered tip 0.009 in. Shaft 0.014 in. 190 and 300 cm length.	Hydrophilic, non-jacketed.	13.3	209
Galeo hydro S	BIOTRONIK	Non-tapered tip. 0.014 in. 175 cm length.	Hydrophilic 12 cm including tip. Hydrophobic shaft. Non-jacketed	3.1	N/A
Galeo hydro F	BIOTRONIK	Non-tapered tip. 0.014 in. 175 cm length.	Hydrophilic 12 cm including tip. Hydrophobic shaft. Non-jacketed	6	N/A
Galeo hydro M	BIOTRONIK	Non-tapered tip. 0.014 in. 175 cm length.	Hydrophilic 12 cm including tip. Hydrophobic shaft. Non-jacketed	4.5	N/A
PT Graphix	Boston	Non-Tapered tip. 0.014 in. 182 and 300 cm lengths	Hydrophilic, non-jacketed.	4.0	26
Shinobi	CORDIS	Non-tapered tip. 0.014 in. 180 and 300 cm lengths	Hydrophillic. Teflon coated.	2.0	13
Shinobi plus	CORDIS	Non-tapered tip. 0.014 in. 180 and 300 cm lengths	Hydrophilic Teflon coated.	4.0	26

Table 3.1 (continued)

Wire	Manufacturer	Design/lengths	Coating	Tip load (g)	Penetration force kg/in.^{2}
Persuader 3	MEDTRONIC	Non-tapered tip. 0.014 in. 190 and 300 cm lengths.	Available in hydrophilic (non-jacketed) and hydrophobic forms. Tip hydrophobic in all variants	5.1	33
Persuader 6	MEDTRONIC	Non-tapered tip. 0.014 in. 190 and 300 cm lengths.	Available in hydrophilic (non-jacketed) and hydrophobic forms. Tip hydrophobic in all variants	8	52
Persuader 9	MEDTRONIC	Tapered tip. 0.010 in., Shaft 0.014 in. 190 and 300 cm lengths.	Available in hydrophilic (non-jacketed) and hydrophobic forms. Tip hydrophobic in all variants	9.1	96
Provia 3	MEDTRONIC	Non-tapered tip. 0.014 in. 180 and 300 cm lengths.	Available in hydrophilic (non-jacketed) and hydrophobic forms. Tip hydrophobic in all variants	3	19
Provia 6	MEDTRONIC	Non-tapered tip. 0.014 in. 180 and 300 cm lengths.	Available in hydrophilic (non-jacketed) and hydrophobic forms. Tip hydrophobic in all variants	6	39

(continued)

Table 3.1 (continued)

Wire	Manufacturer	Design/lengths	Coating	Tip load (g)	Penetration force kg/in.^{2}
Provia 9	MEDTRONIC	Tapered tip. 0.009 in., Shaft 0.014 in. 190 and 300 cm lengths.	Available in hydrophilic (non-jacketed) and hydrophobic forms. Tip hydrophobic in all variants	9	142
Provia 12	MEDTRONIC	Tapered tip. 0.009 in., Shaft 0.014 in. 190 and 300 cm lengths.	Available in hydrophilic (non-jacketed) and hydrophobic forms. Tip hydrophobic in all variants	12	189
Provia 15	MEDTRONIC	Tapered tip. 0.009 in., Shaft 0.014 in. 190 and 300 cm lengths.	Available in hydrophilic (non-jacketed) and hydrophobic forms. Tip hydrophobic in all variants	15	236
Muskie	Vascular Solutions, Inc.	Non-Tapered tip. 0.014 in. 195 and 300 cm lengths.	Hydrophillic, non-jacketed	3	20
Muskie	Vascular Solutions, Inc	Non-tapered tip. 0.014 in. 195 and 300 cm lengths.	Hydrophillic, non-jacketed	4.5	30
Muskie	Vascular Solutions, Inc	Non-tapered tip. 0.014 in. 195 and 300 cm lengths.	Hydrophillic, non-jacketed	6	39
Muskie	Vascular Solutions, Inc	Non-tapered tip. 0.014 in. 195 and 300 cm lengths.	Hydrophillic, non-jacketed	9	58

Table 3.1 (continued)

Wire	Manufacturer	Design/lengths	Coating	Tip load (g)	Penetration force kg/in.^{2}
Muskie	Vascular Solutions, Inc	Non-tapered tip. 0.014 in. 195 and 300 cm lengths.	Hydrophillic, non-jacketed	12	78
High torque floppy extra support	Abbott	Soft tip, high shaft support	Hydrophobic	0.6	N/A
Grand slam	Asahi	Soft tip, high shaft support	Hydrophobic	0.7	N/A
Stabiliser	CORDIS	Soft tip, high shaft support	Hydrophobic	Very soft tip	N/A
Stabiliser plus	CORDIS	Soft tip, very high shaft support	Hydrophobic	Very soft tip	N/A
RG 3	Asahi	Non-tapered tip. Tip 0.014 in., Shaft 0.010 in. 330 cm length	Hydrophilic, non-jacketed over the shaft	3.0	N/A
Rotawire	Boston Scientific	Monofilament wire. Tip 0.014 in. Shaft 0.009 in. 325 cm	Hydrophobic	N/A	N/A
ViperWire advance	Cardiovascular systems	Non-tapered tip. 0.014 in. 330 cm	Hydrophobic	N/A	N/A

N.B. Penetration power is the tip load or tip stiffness (in kg) divided by the area of the wire tip (square inches). It is a better representation of wire penetration ability. Shaft stiffness is a different measure that assesses delivery of equipment along the wire shaft. Penetration efficiency is a new concept in relation to the Gaia wire (Asahi Intecc), which describes the coexistence of high penetration force with maintained steerability and torque response within the CTO segment. Tip load and tip diameter data obtained from the respective manufacturer

crossed, for example because of heavy calcification, wires can be used to enter the wall of the coronary artery. Using wires with slippery coatings attempts can then be made to pass the occluded segment via the subintimal arterial plane, and then to re-enter the lumen distally. Special devices such as the *CrossBoss™* and *Stingray Re-Entry System™* (Boston Scientific, Natick, MA, USA) can help guide a sharp wire back through the vessel wall into the lumen (Fig. 3.2a, b). This technique is called anterograde dissection re-entry (ADR; Case Study 1).

It is sometimes easier to cross an occlusion by entering in a retrograde fashion. Occluded vessels often have well-developed collaterals that supply myocardial territory from another coronary artery. For example, in CTO within the right coronary artery (RCA), distal arterial segments may fill retrogradely via the left anterior descending artery (LAD) septal collaterals. These tiny septals allow the operator to

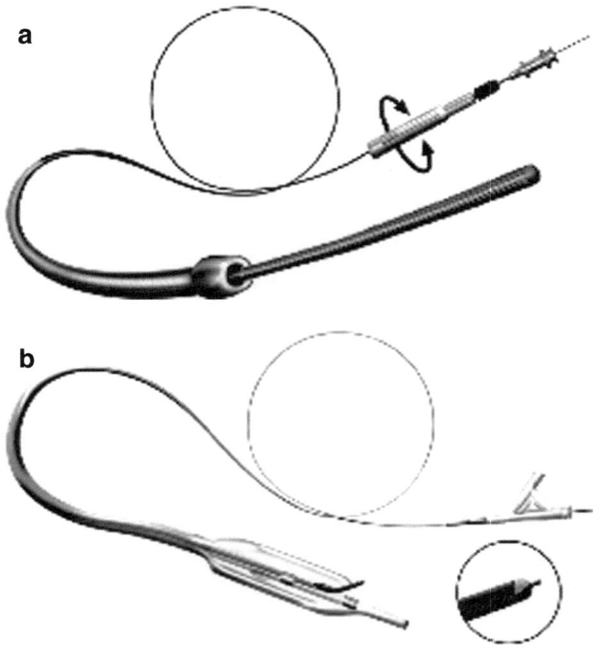

Fig. 3.2 A dedicated dissection/re-entry device – the *CrossBoss™/Stingray Re-Entry System™* (Boston Scientific, Natick, MA, USA). Traversing CTO in the subintimal space requires methods which minimise the risk of perforation. (**a**) The *CrossBoss™* is a metal over the wire microcatheter with a rounded tip allowing safer advancement of wires with high tip stiffness. This catheter is used to traverse the occluded segment through the subintimal space until it is adjacent to normal true lumen where re-entry is attempted. The device is rotated rapidly in a bi-directional manner and advanced without a wire (Image provided courtesy of Boston Scientific. © 2014 Boston Scientific Corporation or its affiliates. All rights reserved). (**b**) The *Stingray device™* facilitates orientation and subsequent successful re-entry into the true lumen. Orientation is via a balloon (*Stingray balloon™*) with two exit ports placed opposite one another and delineated by radio-opaque markers just distally. The balloon assumes a flat shape upon low pressure inflation that is intended to orient one exit port automatically toward the true lumen of the artery. Re-entry using this system uses the *Stingray wire™* which has a high penetration force and an extremely tapered distal tip (Image provided courtesy of Boston Scientific. © 2014 Boston Scientific Corporation or its affiliates. All rights reserved)

approach the RCA CTO from the distal end. Even if the occlusion is crossed in a retrograde fashion, the procedure must finish with anterograde delivery of balloons and stents. Thus two guiding catheters are required, one in the occluded artery and the other in the donor artery (which supplies the collaterals), with the aim of passing a wire from the donor artery through collaterals up into the distal end of the occluded vessel. As with the anterograde approach, the CTO can now be crossed either through the atheroma or by entering the sub-intimal plane to re-enter the proximal lumen. The commonest method is the reverse controlled anterograde and retrograde tracking and dissection (reverse CART) technique (Fig. 3.1b; Case Study 2). If the guidewire can be brought back up into the other guiding catheter it can be exteriorised, a circuit formed (from one guiding catheter, through the coronary circulation, and out of the other guiding catheter), and then balloons and stents successfully delivered anterogradely into the occlusion.

Case Study 1

In 2008, a 68 year old man was treated as an emergency for a non ST elevation myocardial infarction (MI) after 5 months of preceding exertional anginal chest pain. Past medical history included a two vessel CABG in 1996, comprising left internal mammary artery (LIMA) graft to the LAD and saphenous vein graft (SVG) to the RCA. Electrocardiogram (ECG) showed dynamic inferior changes with no regional wall motion abnormality on transthoracic echocardiography (TTE).

Coronary angiography demonstrated mild left main stem artery (LMS) disease, severe long LAD atheroma, 99 % stenosis within a single obtuse marginal (OM) branch of the left circumflex artery (LCx), and an occluded RCA. The LIMA graft was patent but the SVG to RCA graft had a long section of severe atheroma in its mid-course tapering to a 99 % stenosis. PCI was performed to the LCx and SVG graft. A 4 × 30 mm bare metal stent was deployed in the graft and a 2.5 × 80 mm drug eluting stent was implanted within the native vessel.

In October 2012 he was re-admitted as an emergency with a troponin positive acute coronary syndrome. ECG did not show any significant changes. Urgent angiography demonstrated an occlusion proximally just before the previously sited bare metal stent within the right graft. Good collaterals were noted to the distal RCA from the native LCx and his symptoms settled. The patient was discharged on medical therapy including dual anti-platelet agents. Four months later at clinic review, his chest pain had returned allowing an exercise tolerance of only 20 yards. A myocardial perfusion scan (MPS) was requested to look for evidence of objective ischaemia in the RCA territory.

MPS showed extensive inferior wall ischaemia consistent with his occluded native RCA and lack of patent SVG supplying this territory (Fig. 3.3). PCI of the native RCA CTO was discussed and the patient underwent an unsuccessful attempt to re-open the vessel 3 months later. At this first attempt, both anterograde and retrograde techniques were utilised employing specialised wires. However, the dedicated dissection/re-entry device – the *CrossBoss™/Stingray Re-Entry System™* - was unavailable. Two months following this first PCI, a second procedure was undertaken at a different tertiary site using the *CrossBoss™/Stingray Re-Entry System™*, with the additional expertise of a proctor in this method. This second PCI was also unsuccessful but again without complication. Further discussion by all operators led to a uniform agreement that one final attempt be made. This third and final successful procedure took place in April 2014 and was aided by extensive knowledge of the patient's coronary anatomy from the previous two unsuccessful procedures. A repeat anterograde dissection re-entry was performed with a modified re-entry site, and target vessel patency was achieved (Videos 3.1, 3.2, 3.3, 3.4, 3.5, 3.6, 3.7, and 3.8;

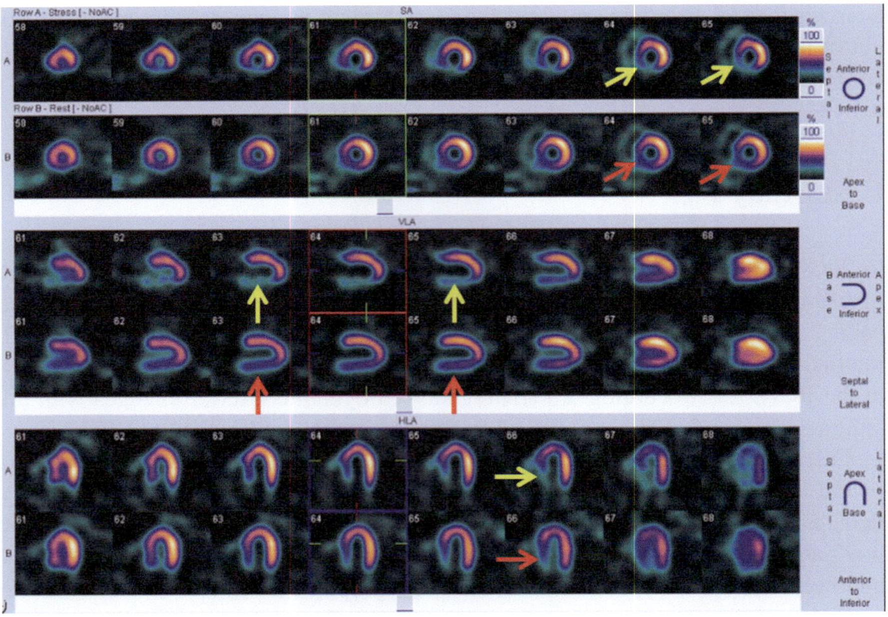

Fig. 3.3 Myocardial perfusion imaging using single-photon emission computed tomography (SPECT). SPECT was performed using physiological stress with technetium-99 m as the radioactive tracer agent. At rest, there was minor reduction in tracer uptake within the basal inferoseptum and basal inferior wall (*red arrows*). Following stress, there was further reduction in tracer uptake - absent uptake at the basal inferior, basal inferoseptal, mid inferior, and apical inferior left ventricular (LV) segments; and moderate reduction within the mid inferoseptum (*yellow arrows*). Summed stress score (SSS) 19 (for low-risk MPS, SSS < 4); automated analysis indicated 21 % of myocardial mass at risk. There was normal LV size and systolic function. In conclusion, MPS demonstrated reversible ischaemia in 5 of 17 myocardial segments, strongly supporting re-vascularisation of the RCA territory

Figs. 3.4 and 3.5). The patient had marked immediate symptomatic improvement, maintained at initial clinic review and at 1 year outpatient follow-up.

Case Study 2

A 47 year old man sustained an inferior MI in 2002. Coronary angiography was not performed at the time of diagnosis. Ten years later, he re-presented as an outpatient with typical anginal symptoms. Diagnostic angiography demonstrated a normal LMS, minor irregularities within the LAD, and a severe proximal stenosis within a large OM branch. The dominant RCA was occluded in the mid-segment with distal filling via antegrade and retrograde collaterals from the left coronary system. This latter lesion was assumed as the culprit for the MI in 2002. Left ventriculography showed inferior hypokinesia, confirmed on TTE. Subsequently, the patient

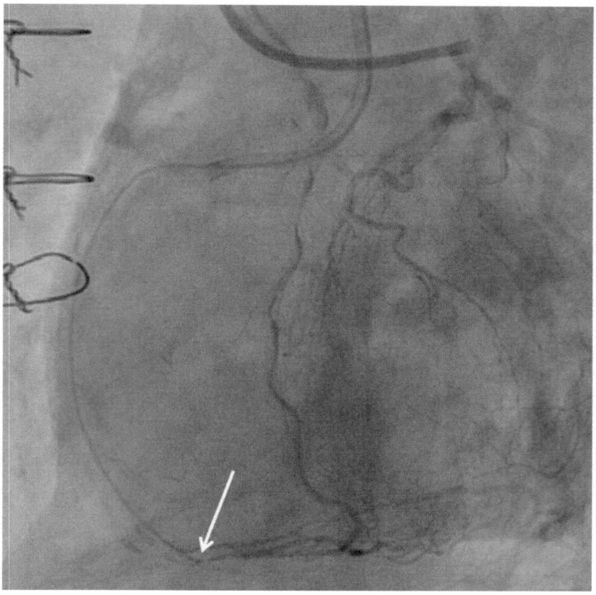

Fig. 3.4 *CrossBoss*™ device in position. Final device position is shown here (*arrowed*)

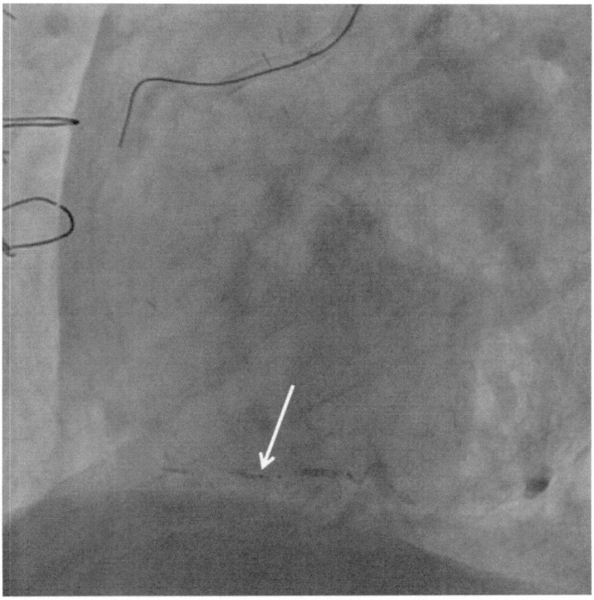

Fig. 3.5 *Stingray balloon*™ in position. Balloon position is shown here (*arrowed*)

underwent PCI and stent implantation to the severe OM stenosis in October 2012. Three weeks after successful intervention, symptoms of exertional dyspnoea and chest discomfort returned prompting urgent repeat angiography which delineated a patent drug-eluting stent. Cardiovascular magnetic resonance (CMR) was requested to assess viability of the inferior myocardial segments (Video 3.9a–f). This was reported as showing good left ventricular (LV) function, with largely scar at the inferior wall, and only minor myocardial ischaemia in the peri-infarct zone. The absence of significant viable myocardium by CMR resulted in continued medical treatment and referral to the gastroenterologists for investigation into a non-cardiac aetiology for the disabling symptoms.

The patient requested a second opinion, which he obtained in December 2013. TTE once again demonstrated hypokinesia of inferior LV segments, specifically basal inferoseptal, and basal to mid inferior walls (Video 3.10a, b). LV ejection fraction was mildly impaired at 50 %. Correlating the significant level of symptoms on optimal medical therapy with the presence of peri-infarct ischaemia on CMR, and the paucity of myocardial damage on TTE despite obstruction in a dominant vessel resulted in attempted PCI of the CTO.

The RCA CTO was successfully re-opened in February 2014 using a retrograde approach – the reverse CART (Videos 3.11, 3.12, 3.13, 3.14, 3.15, and 3.16). Re-canalisation led to a rapid and dramatic reduction of the patient's symptoms (Figs. 3.6, 3.7, 3.8, and 3.9).

Evidence Base for PCI in CTO

Chronic occlusions are found in 20–30 % of all patients with coronary disease investigated by coronary angiography, and their presence is a strong independent predictor of incomplete revascularisation in patients undergoing PCI. In the Synergy between Percutaneous Coronary Intervention with Taxus and Cardiac Surgery (SYNTAX) trial, complete revascularisation was only achieved in 52.8 % of such patients. Successful re-canalisation of a CTO undoubtedly relieves anginal symptoms and a number of observational studies have also reported an association with improved survival. The hypothesis that treatment of CTO by PCI might confer survival advantage is currently being evaluated in two randomised clinical trials, the Drug-Eluting Stent Implantation Versus Optimal Medical Treatment in Patients With Chronic Total Occlusion (DECISION-CTO) trial (NCT01078051) and the European Study on the Utilization of Revascularization versus Optimal Medical Therapy for the Treatment of Chronic Total Coronary Occlusions (EURO-CTO) trial (NCT01760083). These studies are expected to report in 2017.

One way to predict the difficulty of crossing an occlusion is provided by the Multicenter CTO Registry of Japan (J-CTO) score. The score is calculated by assigning 1 point to each of the following five variables: previously failed PCI of the

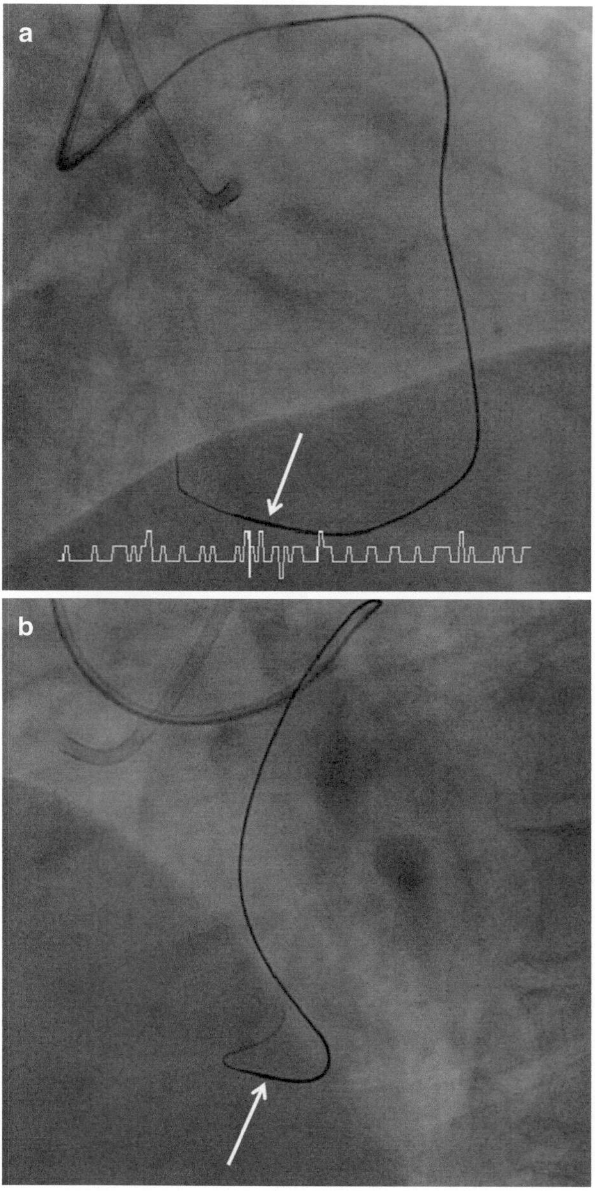

Fig. 3.6 Advancing the *Corsair microcatheter™*. The *Corsair microcatheter™* has now been advanced through the septal collaterals over the retrograde wire. The tip has been marked with an arrow in these views. (**a**) RAO view. (**b**) LAO view

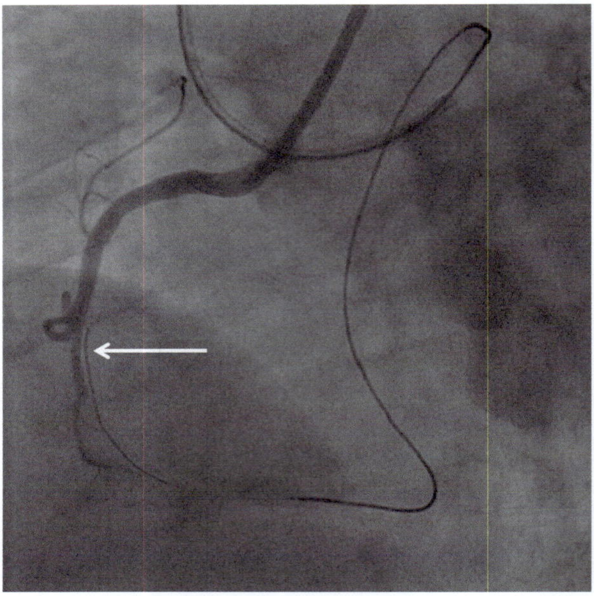

Fig. 3.7 Retrograde wire within the subintimal plane. The retrograde wire has been passed into the subintimal plane, and now sits in the vessel wall alongside the occluded segment (*arrowed*)

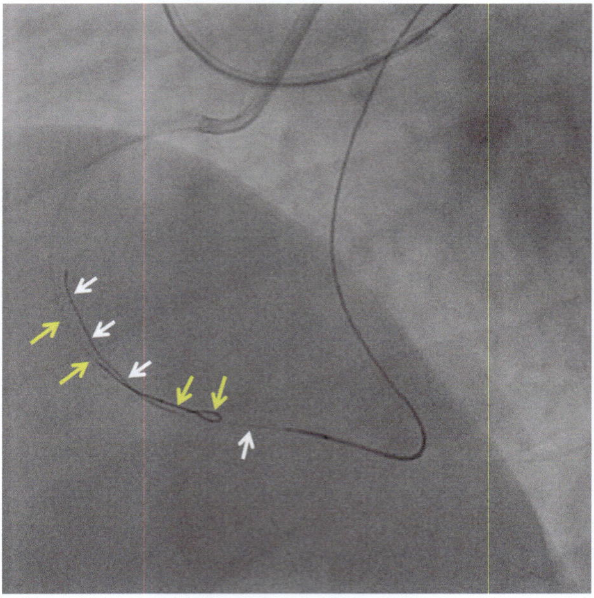

Fig. 3.8 Anterograde wire within the arterial lumen. An anterograde wire has now been passed into the lumen of the occluded RCA. It has then been passed into the subintimal plane and as a 'knuckle' (*yellow arrows*) passes the position of the retrograde wire (*white arrows*), so that both wires now sit adjacent to each other in the subintimal plane

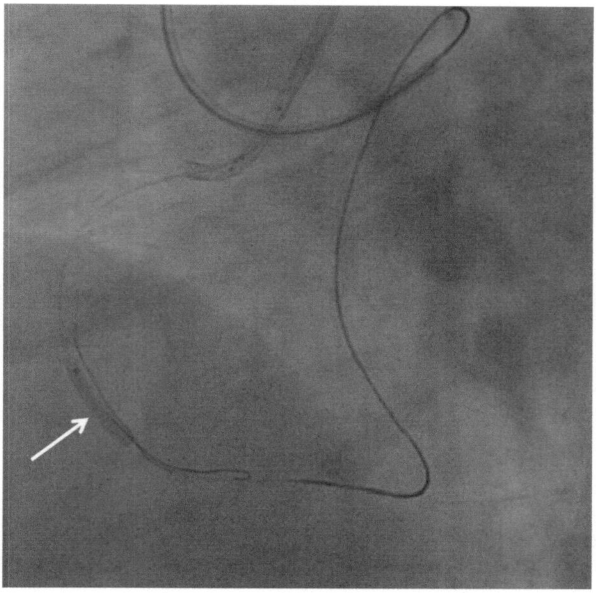

Fig. 3.9 Balloon inflation. A balloon is inflated on the anterograde wire, so creating a space in the subintimal plane (*arrowed*)

lesion, blunt proximal cap, CTO calcification, severe vessel tortuosity, and occlusion length ≥20 mm. Scoring allows classification of patients into four groups: easy (J-CTO score = 0), intermediate (score = 1), difficult (score = 2), and very difficult (score ≥3).

A consistent framework for an optimal strategy to re-canalise a CTO was proposed in 2012 (Fig. 3.10). This provides an overview of the various methods and their application according to four angiographic lesion characteristics:

1. Proximal cap location and morphology
2. Lesion length (dichotomised to < 20 mm versus ≥ 20 mm)
3. Target coronary vessel at distal cap
4. Size and suitability of collateral circulation for retrograde techniques.

Because of the added complexity of these PCI methods, they can be associated with a slightly increased risk of complications compared to more conventional techniques. Procedures may also be more prolonged, thereby increasing the patient's radiation exposure from X-rays. Increased doses of radiographic contrast can increase the risk of contrast induced nephropathy. Increased rates of coronary perforation result from the use of stiff wires required to cross hard fibrocalcific tissue and fine wires traversing delicate collateral channels. Large registries suggest absolute rates of 2.9 % of coronary perforation, 0.3 % resulting in cardiac tamponade, and 3.8 % for contrast nephropathy.

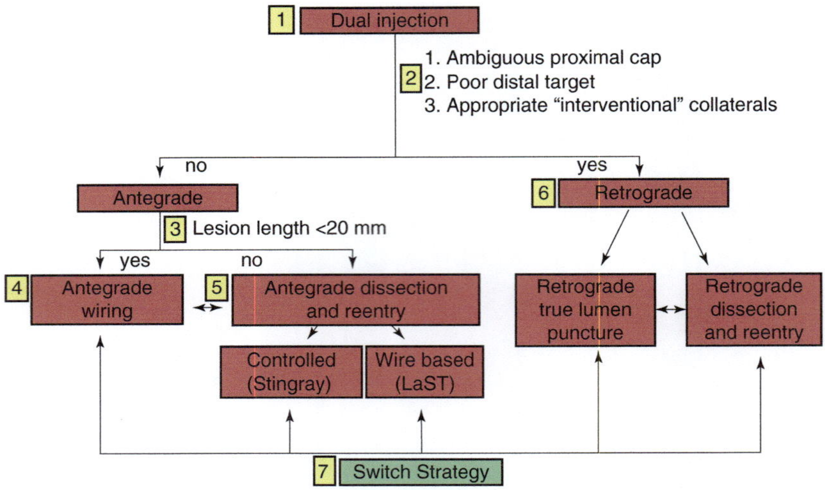

The algorithm starts with dual coronary injection (**box 1**) to allow assessment of several angiographic parameters (**box 2**) and allow selection of a primary antegrade (**boxes 3 to 5**) or primary retrograde (**box 6**) strategy. Strategy changes are made (**box 7**), depending on the progress of the case.
CTO = chronic total occlusion; *LaST* – limited antegrade subintimal tracking

Fig. 3.10 One proposed framework for crossing a CTO by Brilakis et al. [1]

Future of PCI in CTO

Procedural success in CTO PCI ranges between 60–70 % compared with 98 % for other lesion subsets. Recent technological advances and introduction of novel techniques used by specifically trained operators, can improve re-canalisation rates to approximately 90 %. As success rates improve and if survival benefit is confirmed from future trial data, uptake of these advanced PCI techniques will increase. Operator expertise is crucial prior to widespread dissemination. Many interventional centres now allocate only one or two interventional cardiologists to treat CTO at their institution in order to optimise outcomes. Advanced imaging techniques such as CMR assist in decision making prior to undertaking these complex interventions, but the central determinant for attempted PCI in CTO are patient symptoms, and dramatic improvement of pre-existing angina is seen following target vessel re-canalisation.

Recommended Reading

1. Brilakis ES, Grantham JA, Rinfret S et al. A percutaneous treatment algorithm for crossing coronary chronic total occlusions. JACC Cardiovasc Interv. 2012;5:367–79.
2. Brilakis ES, Karmpaliotis D, Werner GS et al. Developments in coronary chronic total occlusion percutaneous coronary interventions: 2014 state-of-the-art update. J Invasive Cardiol. 2014;26:261–6.
3. George S, Cockburn J, Clayton TC et al. Long-term follow-up of elective chronic total coronary occlusion angioplasty: analysis from the u.k. Central cardiac audit database. J Am Coll Cardiol. 2014;64:235–43.

Chapter 4
Percutaneous Management of Mitral Valve Disease

Anitha Varghese, Neal Uren, and Peter F. Ludman

Percutaneous Balloon Valvuloplasty in Mitral Stenosis

Almost all cases of mitral stenosis are due to cardiac disease secondary to rheumatic fever and consequent rheumatic heart disease. Uncommon causes of mitral stenosis include calcification of the mitral valve leaflets and congenital heart disease including a parachute mitral valve. The natural history of rheumatic mitral stenosis is of an asymptomatic latent phase following the initial episode of rheumatic fever. This latent period lasts an average of 16 ± 5 years. Progressive and gradual commissural fusion eventually causes the characteristic symptoms and progression to severe disability may take 9 ± 4 years. Precipitous clinical presentation may occur at the onset of atrial fibrillation causing tachycardia or thromboembolic stroke.

Treatment options for mitral stenosis include medical management, surgical mitral valve replacement (MVR), and percutaneous valvuloplasty using a balloon catheter – percutaneous balloon mitral valvuloplasty (PBMV). Class 1 indications for PBMV are a valve area ≤ 1.5 cm^2 in symptomatic individuals with favourable mitral valve anatomy, or with a contraindication for high risk for surgery. In those offered mitral valve surgery who decline this treatment option, survival on medical therapy alone was 44 ± 6 % at 5 years, and 32 ± 8 % at 10 years after being advised

---

Electronic supplementary material The online version of this chapter (doi:10.1007/978-1-4471-4981-1_4) contains supplementary material, which is available to authorized users.

A. Varghese, MD, MRCP (✉)
London, UK
e-mail: la@doctors.org.uk

N. Uren
Royal Infirmary of Edinburgh, Edinburgh, UK

P.F. Ludman, MA, MD, FRCP
Queen Elizabeth Hospital, Birmingham, UK

A. Varghese et al. (eds.), *Cases in Structural Cardiac Intervention*,
DOI 10.1007/978-1-4471-4981-1_4

surgical correction. To determine which patients would benefit from the percutaneous approach, a scoring system was developed known as the Abascal or Wilkins Echocardiographic Score. Scoring is based on the following 4 echocardiographic criteria:

1. Leaflet mobility,
2. Leaflet thickening,
3. Subvalvar thickening, and
4. Degree of calcification.

Individuals with a score of ≥8 tend to have suboptimal results. A score of <8, a crisp opening snap, and no commissural calcification is associated with excellent procedural outcome.

PBMV is a catheter-based technique that allows mitral valve commisurotomy to be performed in the context of pliable mitral stenosis and has replaced surgery as the favoured approach. PBMV also has an important role in patients with significant mitral stenosis during pregnancy. The stenosed valve is dilated using a specialized balloon – the *Inoue balloon* (Toray Industries Inc; Fig. 4.1). The procedure may be performed under a local anaesthetic, but if transoesophageal echocardiography (TOE) guidance is to be used, then a general anesthetic is preferred (available to view at www.mici.education). A catheter is passed from the right femoral vein to the right atrium. The inter-atrial septum is punctured and the catheter advanced into the left atrium across the septum. A stabilizing wire is positioned within the left atrium over which the Inoue balloon is advanced in its stretched, low-profile configuration,

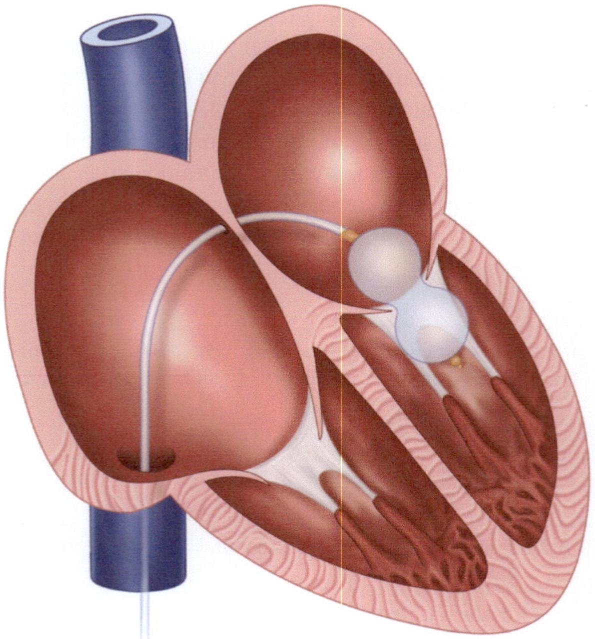

Fig. 4.1 The Inoue balloon. Kanji Inoue, a Japanese Cardiac Surgeon, developed the idea that a degenerated mitral valve could be inflated using a balloon made of strong and pliant natural rubber in 1982. The mechanism and effectiveness of his balloon technique is the same as the abandoned surgical technique of closed mitral commissurotomy

which limits femoral venous and septal punture size. Once positioned in the left atrium, the stretching device is removed, and using a curved stylet the deflated balloon is advanced through the stenosed mitral valve. The Inoue balloon is sub-divided into three segments and is dilated in three stages. First, the distal portion (lying in the left ventricle, LV) is inflated. This portion is pulled gently back against the valve cusps, so preventing the flow of blood pushing the balloon forward and traumatizing the LV apex. As the balloon is further inflated, the second proximal segment dilates thus forming a dumbbell that fixes the central balloon segment exactly at the valve orifice. Finally, as more contrast is introduced into the balloon, the central section inflates to the diameter specified by balloon size, and so splits the mitral valve commissures to relieve the stenosis.

Case Study

A 63 year old lady was referred for consideration of PBMV. She had been fit and well until 2003 when she developed sudden extreme dyspnoea due to the onset of atrial fibrillation (AF) and rapid ventricular response. A diagnosis of mitral stenosis was made on transthoracic echocardiography (TTE) and she responded well to medical therapy, comprising an effective combination of heart rate control, anticoagulation and diuretics. However, over recent years she became progressively more limited by exertional breathlessness, and was in New York Heart Association (NYHA) Class III by the time of referral. Past medical history included diabetes mellitus and the patient could not recall having childhood rheumatic fever. Clinical examination revealed a systolic murmur and loud, rumbling apical diastolic murmur. First heart sound and the pulmonary component of the second heart sound were normal. Jugular venous pressure was not elevated and there was no ankle oedema. Chest was clear. 12-lead electrocardiography showed rate-controlled AF with frequent ventricular ectopy and bigeminy.

Coronary angiography demonstrated no coronary artery disease with a right dominant system and good LV function. No mitral regurgitation was noted at angiography or subsequent TTE evaluation. Pulmonary artery systolic pressure was 55 mmHg with a mean of 28 mmHg. In-patient TOE assessment was organized prior to PBMV (Videos 4.1, 4.2, and 4.3). Due to the finding of left atrial appendage thrombus, the planned procedure was deferred for 6 months until the clot resolved after increased anti-thrombotic medication. At peri-procedural TOE several months later, severe mitral stenosis was confirmed (Figs. 4.2a–d; Video 4.4). PBMV was then successfully performed (Videos 4.5, 4.6, 4.7, 4.8, and 4.9).

With careful pre-procedural patient selection, PBMV is associated with excellent success rates and low rate of complications. The most serious adverse event is the occurrence of acute severe mitral regurgitation, usually resulting from a tear in one of the valve leaflets or the subvalvular apparatus. This complication can lead to pulmonary oedema and hemodynamic compromise, necessitating urgent surgical MVR. Other serious complications during PBMV usually relate to the transseptal

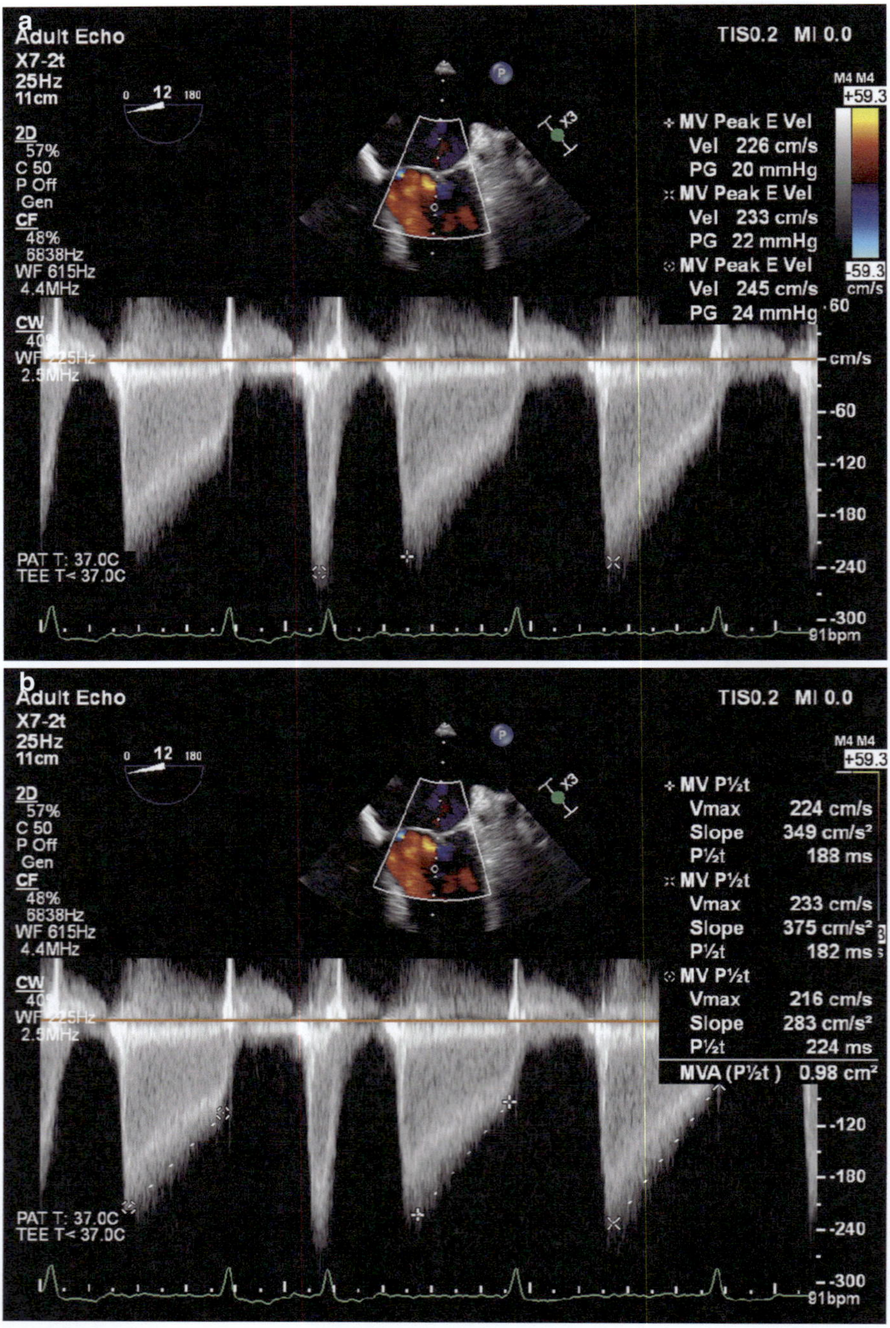

Fig. 4.2 Echocardiographic assessment mitral stenosis severity. (**a**) Continuous wave Doppler through the stenosed valve confirming a high instantaneous peak velocity, corresponding to a peak gradient of 22 mmHg. (**b**) Mitral valve area measured by pressure half time of 0.98 cm^2. (**c**) Velocity time integral analysis showed a mean gradient of approximately 12 mmHg. (**d**) Three-dimensional planimetry demonstrated a mitral valve area of 1.1 cm^2

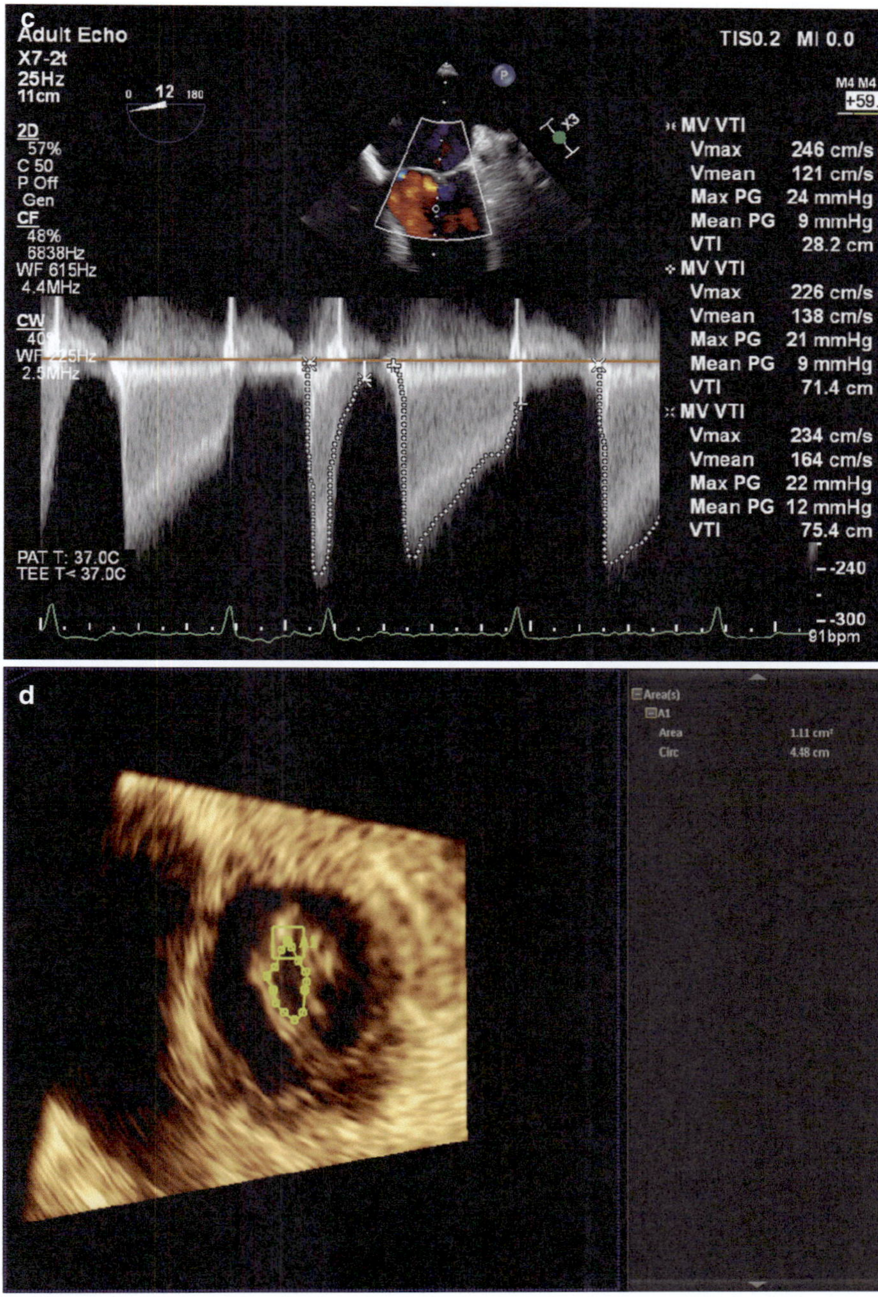

Fig. 4.2 (continued)

puncture. The ideal site for puncture is at the region of the fossa ovalis. Occasionally, the sharp needle can inadvertently traumatize other cardiac structures leading to cardiac tamponade or serious blood loss.

PBMV does not provide permanent relief from mitral stenosis. Regular follow-up is mandatory to detect re-stenosis in this patient cohort. Up to 70–75 % of individuals can remain free of re-stenosis 10 years following the procedure, but this number falls to about 40 % 15 years post valvuloplasty.

Percutaneous Mitral Valve Repair in Mitral Regurgitation

Mitral regurgitation can be caused by degenerative valve disease (mitral valve prolapse in 20–50 % of cases), or heart muscle disease (13–30 %), rheumatic heart disease (3–20 %), endocarditis (10–12 %) or, rarely, congenital heart disease. These causes may be grouped into three main descriptive categories:

1. Functional regurgitation (both ischaemic and non-ischaemic)
2. Degenerative regurgitation (mitral valve prolapse)
3. Other causes (including post-rheumatic, post-endocardits, congenital).

In patients with functional mitral regurgitation, whether associated with ischaemic or non-ischemic heart disease (i.e. dilated cardiomyopathy), the valve leaflets are intrinsically normal but leaflet mobility is restricted due to displacement of the papillary muscles, in turn due to LV dilatation and/or dilatation of the valve annulus. In contrast, degenerative mitral valve disease is characterised by myxomatous degeneration of the valve leaflets and changes in the sub-valvular apparatus including stretching and/or rupture of the chordae tendineae.

Patients with severe symptomatic mitral regurgitation have a poor prognosis with an annual mortality rate of 5 % per year without surgical intervention. Mitral valve surgery (repair or replacement) is the second commonest valve operation performed in the developed world according to figures reported to the Society for Thoracic Surgeon (STS) Database in 2002. Patients with severe mitral regurgitation with evidence of LV dysfunction or dilatation are currently recommended for surgery whether they are symptomatic or not. If considered too high risk for surgery, a percutaneous option to mitral valve repair is sometimes possible. The most established system of repair is an edge-to-edge reconstruction while the heart is beating - the *MitraClip® system* (Abbott Vascular, CA, USA; Fig. 4.3a–c).

Case Study

A complete case study in video format is available to view at www.mici.education. As shown, the MitraClip® procedure is performed in the cardiac catheterisation laboratory with TOE and fluoroscopic guidance while the patient is under general

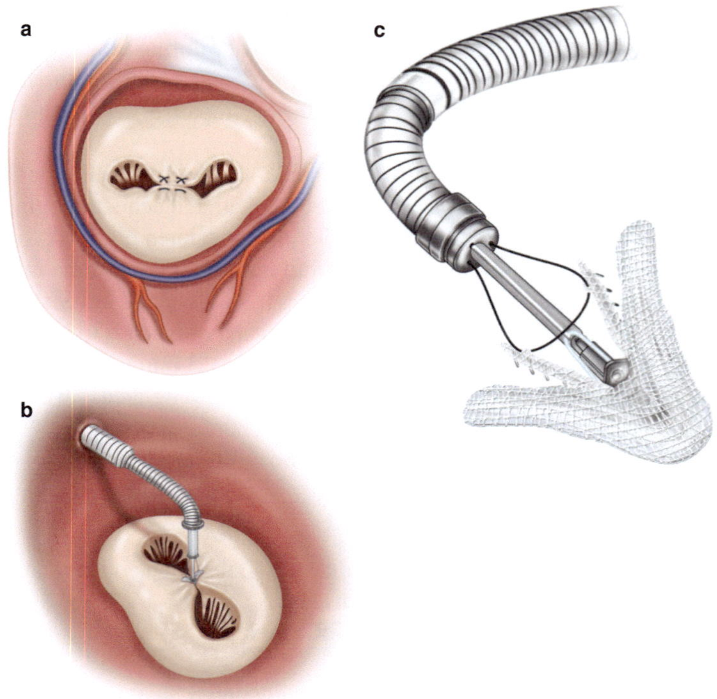

Fig. 4.3 Edge-to-edge reconstruction technique. (**a**) Surgical repair. The edge-to-edge repair has been used as a surgical technique in open chest arrested heart surgery for the treatment of mitral regurgitation since the early 1990s, and is known as the "Alfieri Technique" after its progenitor. A portion of the anterior leaflet is sutured to the corresponding portion of the posterior leaflet creating a point of permanent coaptation ("approximation") of the two leaflets. When the edge-to-edge suture is placed in the middle of the valve, the valve will have a functional double orifice during diastole, hence the alternate name of the "Double Orifice Repair". The valve can still open on both sides of the suture, allowing adequate diastolic blood flow through the valve. The suture assures that the two leaflets come together properly, as required, during systole. Tissue approximation is increasingly maintained over time by the healing response that takes place between the sutured leaflets, gradually reducing the need for the mechanical support provided by the stitches. The Alfieri surgical repair has been successfully used with mid-term follow-up to treat all of the primary (degenerative) aetiologies of mitral regurgitation. The new valve geometry resulting from edge-to-edge repair will have a smaller effective diastolic orifice size than prior to the procedure, just as is expected after valve repair with adjunctive annuloplasty or after valve replacement. A normal mitral valve has an effective diastolic orifice area of around 6.0 cm^2. The edge-to-edge repair technique typically reduces the effective diastolic orifice area by 40–50 %, without associated significant valvular diastolic pressure gradient or stenosis over time. In the majority of edge-to-edge procedures, most surgeons insert an annuloplasty ring at the time of index surgery even if the mitral valve annulus is not significantly dilated in order to reduce the likelihood of re-operation. (**b** and **c**) *MitraClip® system*. (**b**) An atrial view of the deployed device grasping both leaflets of the mitral valve. As is evident, this percutaneous system is based on the surgical Alfieri procedure. The aim is to create a competent double orifice valve by suturing the free edges of the middle part of the anterior mitral valve leaflet (A2) to the corresponding part of the posterior valve leaflet (P2). (**c**) The device comprises a cobalt-chromium alloy covered with polypropylene fabric which promotes tissue in-growth. A single size clip has been used to treat patients with functional, mixed and degenerative mitral regurgitation. A dual-arm structure with grippers above the arms assists leaflet capture and approximation on the beating heart

anaesthesia. It has been suggested that the identification of the optimum point for creating the edge-to-edge repair of the leaflets is easier during a beating heart procedure. This is not possible with surgical repair, which can result in the need to re-initiate cardio pulmonary bypass to perform further repair or MVR should repair fail. Multiple clips can be positioned.

Key to procedural success is the pre-assessment of valve suitability for the percutaneous approach. Assessment requires detailed clinical and echocardiographic data interpretation in cases of severe mitral regurgitation considered high risk for surgery. The primary regurgitant jet should originate from mal-coaptation of the mitral valve in a location accessible by the *MitraClip® device*. If a secondary jet exists, it should be considered clinically insignificant. Certain leaflet anatomy leads to less successful implantation, such as a flail segment width greater than 15 mm or a flail gap greater than 10 mm, evidence of calcification or cleft at the grasping area, severe bi-leaflet prolapse, and a lack of both primary and secondary chordal support.

The following exclusion criteria should also be considered:

- Severe mitral annular calcification.
- Prior mitral valve leaflet surgery.
- Echocardiographic evidence of intracardiac mass, thrombus or vegetation.
- Active endocarditis or rheumatic heart disease.
- Active infections requiring current antibiotic therapy.
- Patients where TOE is contraindicated.
- Presence of a permanent pacemaker or pacing leads that may interfere with placement of the device.

The Evidence Base for a Percutaneous Approach

The *MitraClip® system* was evaluated in two landmark clinical trials in 47 US and Canadian centres: EVEREST (Endovascular Valve Edge-to-Edge Repair Study) I and EVEREST II.

EVEREST I was a feasibility trial in 55 patients of median age 71 years with a median LV ejection fraction (LVEF) of 62 %, 46 % of whom were NYHA Class III or IV. In this study group, along with 60 patients from the roll-in phase of EVEREST II, the 30-day freedom from clinical events was 91 %, with one non-clip-related death, one stroke after 72 hours, two requiring surgery for transseptal complications, and four requiring more than two units blood transfusion. At 12 months, 92 % of patients were in NYHA Class I-II; 77 % showed an improvement in NYHA class, 17 % had no change, and 6 % were worse. In terms of LV remodelling, there was a significant reduction in LV end-diastolic volume (LVEDV) from 174 to 151 ml and in LV end-systolic volume (LVESV) from 72 to 64 ml in all patients. In those with LV dysfunction (LVEF<55 %), the LVEDV fell from 207 to 171 ml, and the LVESV from 109 to 86 ml. At 3 years follow-up, 96 % of patients were still alive with 82 % free from cardiac surgery with no mitral stenosis reported after 2 years of follow-up.

EVEREST II was the first randomised trial of any minimally invasive mitral valve repair device compared to surgical valve repair or replacement. A total of 279 patients were randomly assigned to *MitraClip®* *versus* surgery in a 2:1 ratio. The primary safety endpoint of any major adverse event was significantly lower in the *MitraClip®* treated patients compared to surgery (9.6 % MitraClip patients versus 57 % surgical patients). The primary effectiveness endpoint (freedom from death, re-do surgery or residual significant mitral regurgitation) of the *MitraClip® device* was non-inferior to surgery at 1 year. There was a highly significant reduction in the severity of mitral regurgitation in the *MitraClip®* treated patients. Overall, 81.5 % of patients improved to mild or moderate mitral regurgitation from a severe category with LV diastolic volume falling by 13 %. Patients' symptoms improved following a successful *MitraClip®* procedure. At baseline, 52.6 % of patients had moderate or severe symptoms (NYHA Class III or IV), while at 1 year 97.5 % had no or only mild symptoms (NYHA Class I or II). There was also a highly significant improvement in patients' quality of life assessed using the SF-36 survey. Four year follow-up of the EVEREST II trial confirmed similar mortality in both groups, 17.4 % and 17.8 % in the *MitraClip®* and surgery groups respectively with similar rates of 3+ or 4+ mitral regurgitation (22–25 %). In the *MitraClip®* group, 25 % required subsequent surgery compared to 6 % in the surgery group at 4 years (the majority of which occurred in the first year of follow-up).

An additional 78 patients were included in an EVEREST II high-risk registry. In this registry, the 30-day mortality was reported at 7.7 % (no procedure-related deaths) compared to an estimated mortality of 18.2 % had the patients undergone conventional mitral valve surgery. Furthermore, at 30 days, 82 % of patients had mitral regurgitation of 2+ or less which was sustained out to 1 year follow-up in parallel with an improvement in symptoms. This benefit in high-risk patients with functional mitral regurgitation was confirmed in an observational trial of 50 patients with severe heart failure (LVEF<25 %; mean EuroSCORE 34 %) with 72 % of patients achieving NYHA Class I or II at 6 months associated with concomitant reductions in LV volume and measures of heart failure (pro N-Terminal brain natriuretic peptide levels). A recent meta-analysis of one randomised trial (EVEREST II) and three prospective observational studies confirmed complete non-inferiority between *MitraClip®* and surgery with regard to 1 year mortality, neurological events, need for re-operation for failed procedures, and NYHA class, with only residual mitral regurgitation severity>2+ being higher in the *MitraClip®* group (17 % versus 0.4 %). The *MitraClip®* patients were older with lower LVEF and higher EuroSCOREs. In a recent European post-approval registry of *MitraClip®* therapy, 567 patients (mean logistic EuroSCORE 23 ± 18 %) underwent the procedure with

3.4 % 30-day and 18.2 % 1 year mortality. A total of 6.3 % required mitral valve surgery within a year of the procedure with 71 % NYHA Class I or II.

Future of Percutaneous Mitral Valve Intervention

PBMV is an established and effective technique in selected cases of mitral stenosis. Advances in imaging will continue to support the success of this important therapy. However, the mechanisms that cause mitral regurgitation are numerous and complex, involving not only the valve and its chordae but also ventricular anatomy and annular dimensions. Surgical approaches often combine multiple techniques to address all these aspects, but percutaneous techniques are still in their infancy and a variety of different approaches are under investigation.

Recommended Reading

1. Abascal VM, Wilkins GT, O'Shea JP et al. Prediction of successful outcome in 130 patients undergoing percutaneous balloon mitral valvotomy. Circulation. 1990;82(2):448–56.
2. Feldman T, Wasserman HS, Herrmann HC et al. Percutaneous mitral valve repair using the edge-to-edge technique: six-month results of the EVEREST Phase I Clinical Trial. J Am Coll Cardiol. 2005;46:2134–40.
3. Maisano F, Franzen O, Baldus S et al. Percutaenous mitral valve interventions in the real world: early and one-year results from the ACCESS-EU, a prospective, multicenter non-randomised post-approval study of the Mitraclip therapy in Europe. J Am Coll Cardiol. 2013;62(12):1052–61.
4. Nobuyoshi M, Arita T, Shirai S, Hamasaki N, Yokoi H, Iwabuchi M, Yasumoto H, Nosaka H. Percutaneous balloon mitral valvuloplasty – a review. Circulation. 2009;119:e211–9.
5. Wan B, Rahnavardi M, Tian DH, Phan K, Munkholm-Larsen S, Bannon PG, Yan TD. A meta-analysis of Mitraclip system versus surgery for treatment of severe mitral regurgitation. Ann Cardiothorac Surg. 2013;2(6):683–92.
6. Wilkins GT, Weyman AE, Abascal VM, Block PC, Palacios IF. Percutaneous balloon dilatation of the mitral valve: an analysis of echocardiographic variables related to outcome and the mechanism of dilatation. Heart. 1988;60(4):299–308.

Chapter 5
Percutaneous Paravalvular Leak Closure

Anitha Varghese, Neal Uren, and Peter F. Ludman

Paravalvular regurgitation affects 5–17 % of all surgically implanted prosthetic heart valves. Patients who have paravalvular regurgitation can be asymptomatic or present with symptoms arising from ongoing haemolysis or heart failure. Re-operation is associated with increased morbidity and is not always successful because of underlying tissue friability, inflammation or calcification. Percutaneous paravalvular leak closure is now an established therapy for symptomatic patients (Fig. 5.1a, b; available to view at www.mici.education). Comprehensive echocardiographic imaging with transthoracic echocardiography (TTE) and three-dimensional transoesophageal echocardiography (3D TOE) is key in characterizing defect location, size and shape. For para-mitral defects, an anterograde transseptal approach can be performed successfully guided by biplane fluoroscopy and 3D TOE (Fig. 5.2a–h). Alternative approaches to such defects include retrograde transaortic cannulation or transapical access and retrograde cannulation (Fig. 5.3a, b). For oblong or crescentic defects, the simultaneous or sequential deployment of two smaller devices as opposed to one large device results in a higher degree of procedural success and safety because the risk of impingement on the prosthetic leaflets is minimized. Most para-aortic defects can be approached in a retrograde manner and closed with a single device (Fig. 5.4a–k). With careful anatomical assessment, procedural planning and execution, successful closure rates of 90 % or more are

---

Electronic supplementary material The online version of this chapter (doi:10.1007/978-1-4471-4981-1_5) contains supplementary material, which is available to authorized users.

A. Varghese, MD, MRCP (✉)
London, UK
e-mail: la@doctors.org.uk

N. Uren
Royal Infirmary of Edinburgh, Edinburgh, UK

P.F. Ludman, MA, MD, FRCP
Queen Elizabeth Hospital, Birmingham, UK

A. Varghese et al. (eds.), *Cases in Structural Cardiac Intervention*,
DOI 10.1007/978-1-4471-4981-1_5

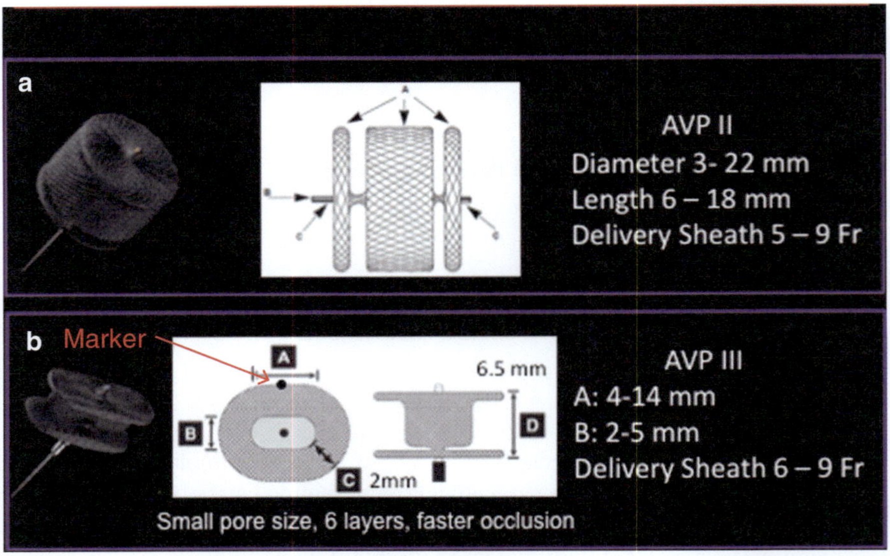

Fig. 5.1 *Amplatzer™ Vascular Plug* (AVP; St. Jude Medical, Inc., Plymouth, MN). (**a**) AVP II and (**b**) AVP III. These devices are made of self-expanding finely braided nitinol wire mesh. A device is selected according to the dimensions and shape of the defect to be occluded. The AVP II is more suited to circular defects, whereas the oblong shape of the AVP III fits well in the more slit like and crescentic holes (AMPLATZER and St. Jude Medical are trademarks of St. Jude Medical, Inc. or its related companies. Reproduced with permission of St. Jude Medical, © 2016. All rights reserved)

attainable with a low risk of device impingement on the prosthetic valve or embolization.

The therapeutic endpoint should be determined before initiating the procedure. If the procedure is being done primarily for treatment of heart failure, any marked reduction in regurgitant volume is likely to help the patient. However, if the procedure is done primarily to treat haemolysis, complete obliteration of regurgitation is usually necessary for efficacy. Important considerations clearly include determining which specific leak is responsible for the haemolysis. Should residual regurgitation be present, color flow Doppler assessment can be extremely difficult because of splaying of the jet through the residual leak and around the first device. Measuring left atrial pressure does not usually help because pressure typically does not decrease immediately.

Tilting-disk valves may be pulled shut during device deployment, which can be recognised immediately if the fluoroscopic planes are set up correctly. Valve obstruction may be relieved by reversing the deployment manoeuvre and pushing the delivery catheter and device back into the mid left ventricle (LV). Devices may also obstruct prosthetic valve leaflets during systole and prevent valve closure. In this scenario, frequently the only sign is an abrupt increase in valvular regurgitation that is greater than the normal closing volume. Rarely, a device may tilt after deployment and block the prosthetic leaflet. If this occurs, two options are available. The first is to use a long, flexible, bioptome through the steerable left atrial sheath. The second option is to snare the distal portion of the device and pull it anterograde through the defect. Failure of these manoeuvres will necessitate surgery. Stroke or transient ischemic attacks can result from systemic thromboembolism, either peri- or post-procedure and are related to transition of anticoagulation regimens. Therefore meticulous attention to catheter flushing and adequate heparinisation are mandatory.

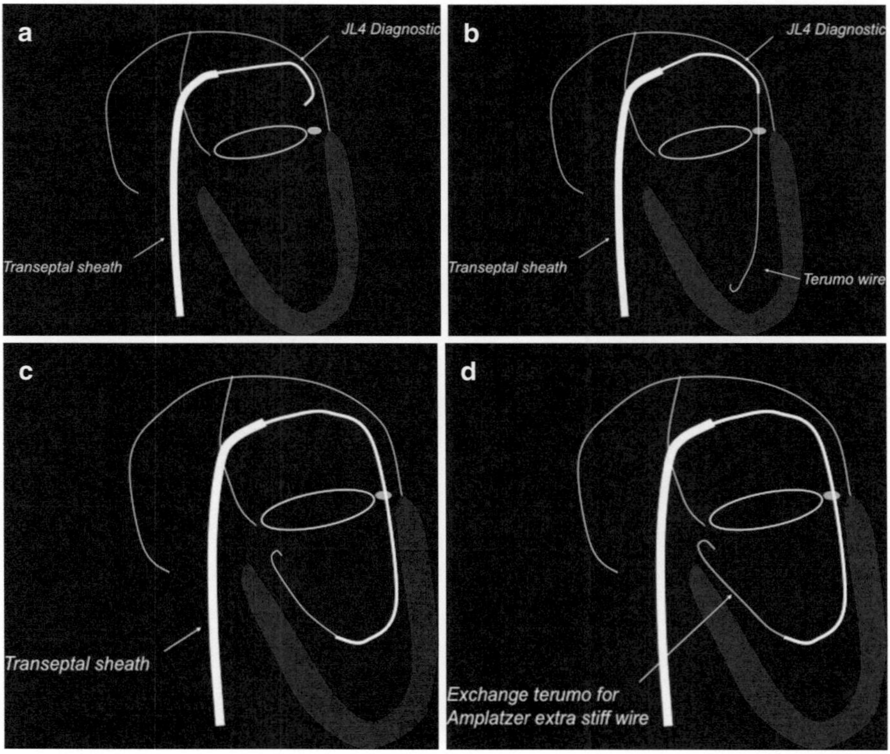

Fig. 5.2 Anterograde, transseptal approach to close a mitral paravalvular leak. (**a**) A transseptal sheath has been placed in position across the inter-atrial septum, and a left Judkins coronary diagnostic catheter is introduced. (**b**) A *Terumo*™ *guide wire* (Terumo Europe NV) is guide wire is advanced through the Judkins catheter and manipulated so as to cross the defect into the left ventricle (LV). (**c**) The Judkins catheter is advanced over the wire to follow it into the LV. (**d**) The *Terumo*™ *wire* is removed and replaced with an *Amplatz*™ *extra stiff wire* (Cook Medical), to provide a more rigid rail. (**e**) A delivery sheath is advanced over the stiff wire across the defect. (**f**) The closure device is introduced through the delivery sheath. (**g**) The distal disc of the closure device is advanced out of the sheath, and as it does so the nitinol frame conforms to its original unconstrained shape. (**h**) The device is pulled back so that the distal disc sits on the ventricular side of the defect. As the delivery sheath is pulled further back the proximal disc is released from constraint and also assumes its original shape on the atrial side of the defect. Careful assessment is then carried out to check that the device is securely in position and that the discs are not obstructing the mitral valve leaflets. The delivery cable is subsequently detached from the device and the equipment withdrawn leaving the closure device in place

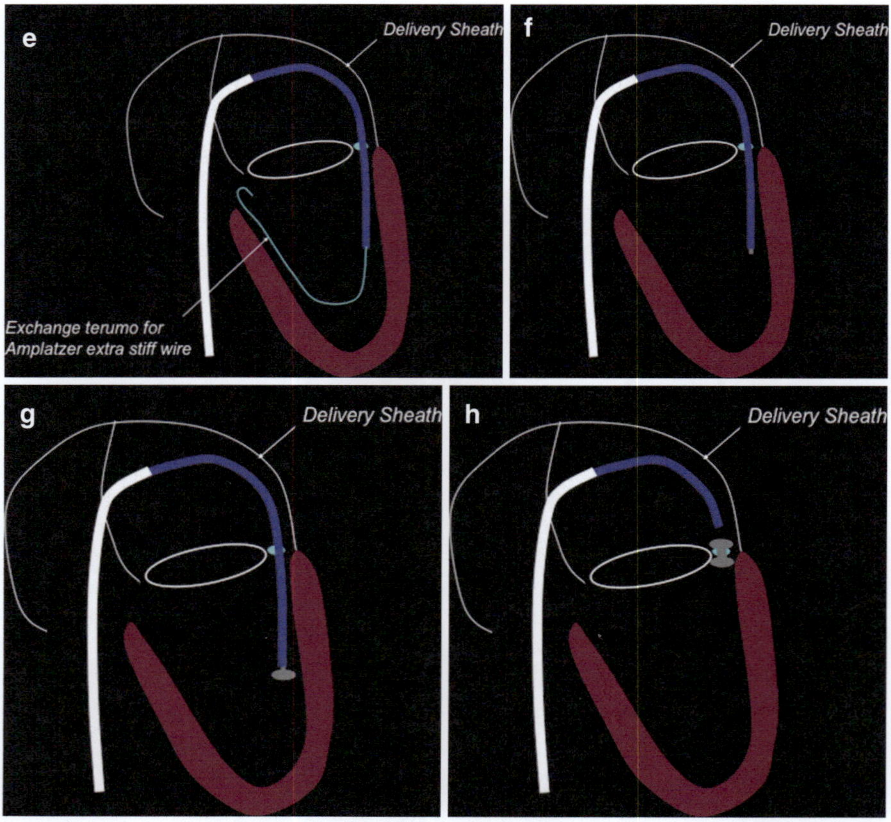

Fig. 5.2 (continued)

Para-Mitral Valve Prosthesis Leak Closure

Para-mitral defects account for 80 % of cases. The standard clock-face view used by echocardiographers to describe the mitral valve ring is left-right reversed compared to the traditional left atrial surgical view and close communication between echocardiographer and interventionalist is required (Fig. 5.5). When differentiation of transvalvular and paravalvular regurgitation is difficult, intracardiac echocardiography (ICE) may be used. The anterograde trans septal approach is the commonest technique used (Fig. 5.6a, b). Occasionally, if a defect is medial and difficult to access transseptally, a transapical approach is preferred.

An alternative method is to deploy the devices sequentially ((Fig. 5.7a–c). In this approach, a hydrophilic guidewire is snared and exteriorised. All catheters are removed and replaced with an 8F sheath. With the arteriovenous (AV) guidewire rail

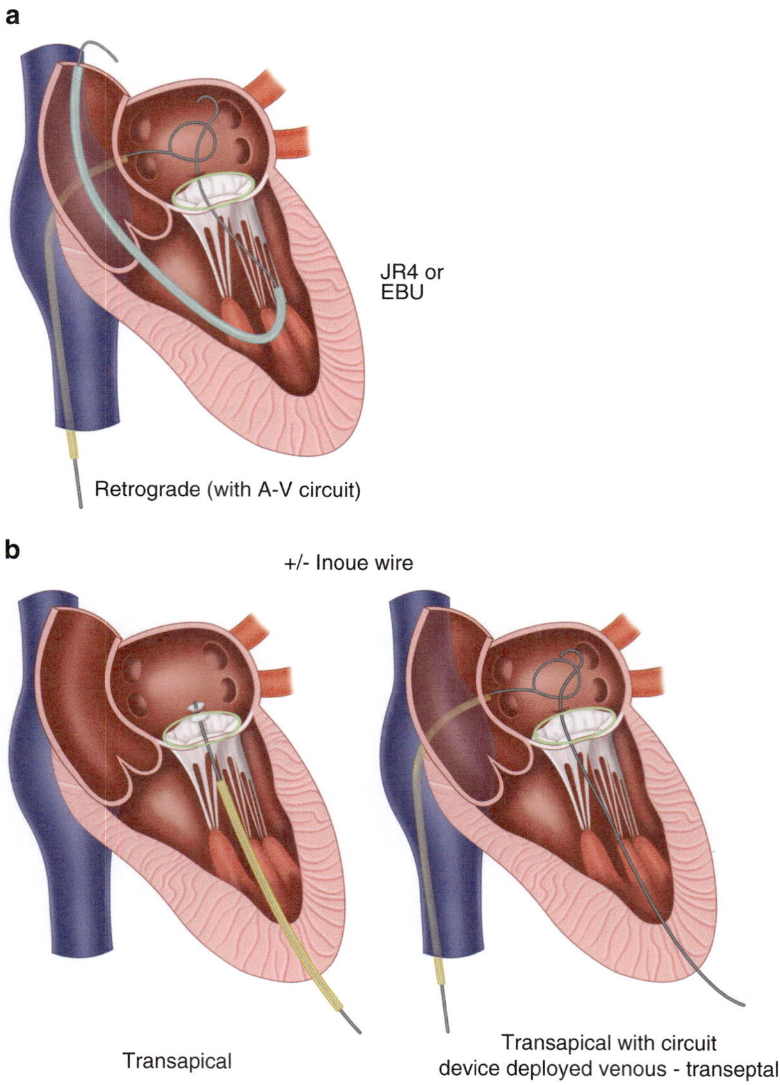

Fig. 5.3 Alternative approaches to mitral paravalvular leak closure. (**a**) An example of a retrograde approach. A wire has been passed retrogradely from the femoral artery to the aortic root, and across the aortic valve to the LV. A Judkins shaped or extra back-up shaped catheter is used to help steer the wire back through the paravalvular defect and into the left atrium. A transseptal catheter is passed from the femoral vein to the right atrium and across the inter-atrial septum to the left atrium. This is used to introduce a snare to capture the retrograde wire. A 'circuit' can then be created from the femoral artery, through the defect and back out to the femoral vein. This circuit is used to introduce a delivery sheath and deploy a device in the defect. (**b**) A transapical approach. The apex of the LV is punctured through the anterior chest wall, and a wire introduced into the ventricle. From here it is directed retrogradely across the defect into the left atrium. A delivery catheter is then placed over this wire and an occlusion device delivered to the defect. If the defect is large, the delivery sheath required may be of a large diameter. To avoid creating a large puncture in the LV apex, an anterograde approach might be favoured. For this method the wire is snared in the left atrium, and a circuit created. The large delivery sheath can then be introduced through the femoral vein and the occluder delivered in an anterograde fashion

in position, the first closure device can be placed through this sheath, alongside the existing guidewire rail. After placement of the first device, the sheath is removed from over the delivery cable of the first device and then replaced over the existing loop of the AV guidewire rail, leaving the first device tethered on its cable. A second, or even third, device can then be placed with use of similar techniques. After efficacy and prosthetic valve leaflet function are assured by 3D TOE and fluoroscopy, all devices can be released. The sequential technique is particularly useful for very large paravalvular defects (about 25 % of the sewing ring) which can be closed more effectively with staggered "nesting" of the devices.

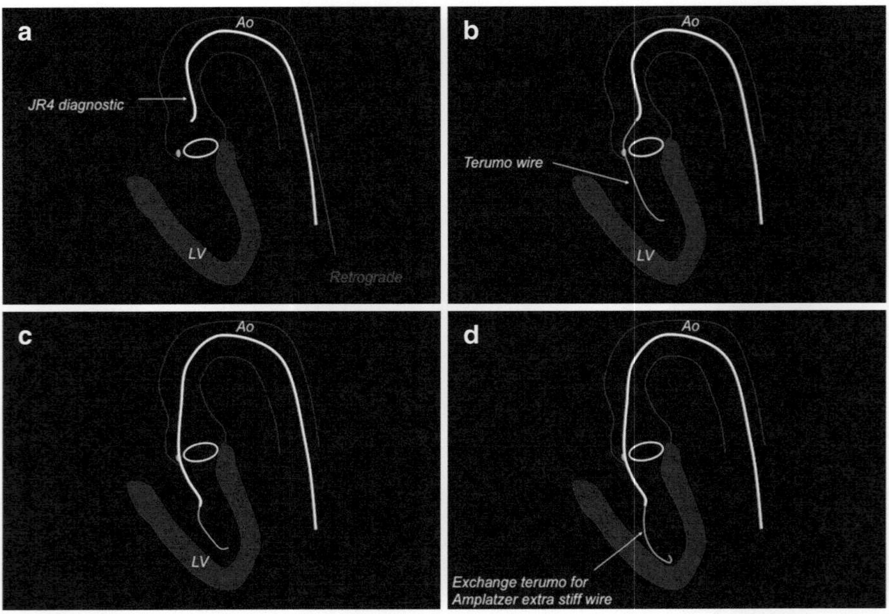

Fig. 5.4 Retrograde approach to aortic paravalvular leak closure. (**a**) A Judkins diagnostic catheter is introduced to the aortic root. (**b**) A *Terumo*™ wire is used through this catheter to cross the defect. (**c**) The catheter follows the wire into the LV. (**d**) The *Terumo*™ wire is switched for the more supportive *Amplatz*™ *extra stiff* wire. (**e**) The catheter is withdrawn. (**f**) A delivery sheath is introduced on the stiff wire, across the defect. (**g**) The closure device is advanced attached to the delivery cable. (**h**) The distal disc is released to adopt its normal configuration. (**i**) The distal disc is pulled back against the LV side of the defect. (**j**) The proximal disc is released. (**k**) Checks are made to ensure device stability and that there is no interference with valve function, and then it is released from its delivery cable

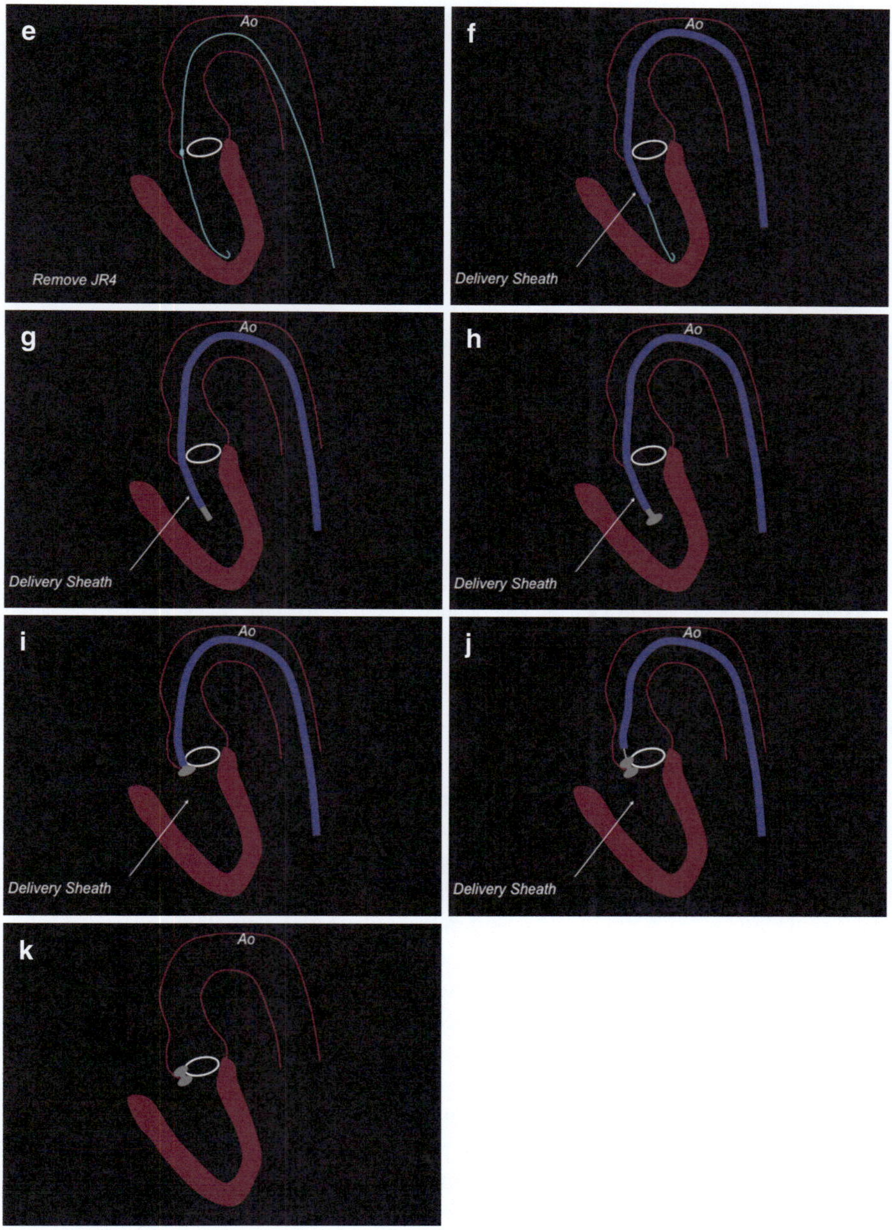

Fig. 5.4 (continued)

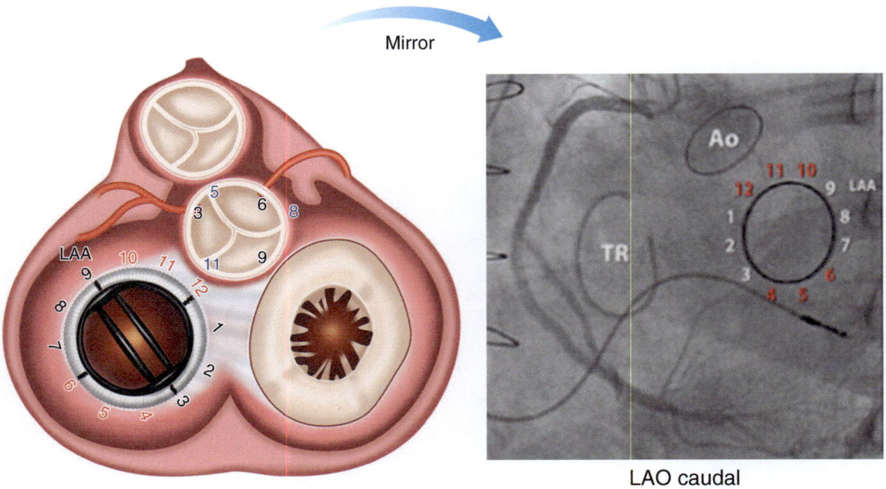

Fig. 5.5 Comparison of transoesophageal echocardiographic and angiographic imaging. On the left side is a representation of the usual alignment of the echocardiographic image, called the 'surgeon's view', with the left atrial appendage top left. On the right, is the view obtained using fluoroscopy, camera positioned in a left anterior oblique (LAO) with caudal angulation. *LAA* left atrial appendage, *LAO* left anterior oblique view, *Ao* aorta, *TR* tricuspid valve annuloplasty ring

Case Study: Mitral Position

A 77 year old was referred for consideration of either percutaneous or surgical closure of para-mitral valve leaks. She had a background of rheumatic heart disease. Bioprosthetic aortic and mitral valve replacements were implanted in 1980, 31 years previously. Re-do cardiac surgery was required in 1991, and the bioprostheses were replaced by mechanical aortic and mitral valves using single disc Bjork-Shiley valves. Seventeen years following re-operation, investigations for flu-like symptoms revealed a severe haemolytic anaemia resulting from paravalvular leak of the mechanical mitral valve. Despite multiple and regular blood transfusions (two units of blood every 2 weeks) haemoglobin levels continued to fall. The patient was effectively housebound with New York Heart Association (NYHA) Class IV symptoms. She was jaundiced and frail and a percutaneous approach was agreed after multidisciplinary review and discussion with the patient.

Towards the end of 2010, she was admitted for attempted paravalvular leak closure. TOE demonstrated severe mitral regurgitation due to two para-mitral leaks close to the atrial septum in a postero-medial position. Warfarin anticoagulation was converted to intravenous heparin. She was in atrial fibrillation and ventricular function was preserved. The first closure attempt was made anterogradely using transseptal puncture. While it was possible to cross one of the defects using the wire, the sheath could not be advanced and the procedure was abandoned. One week later, a

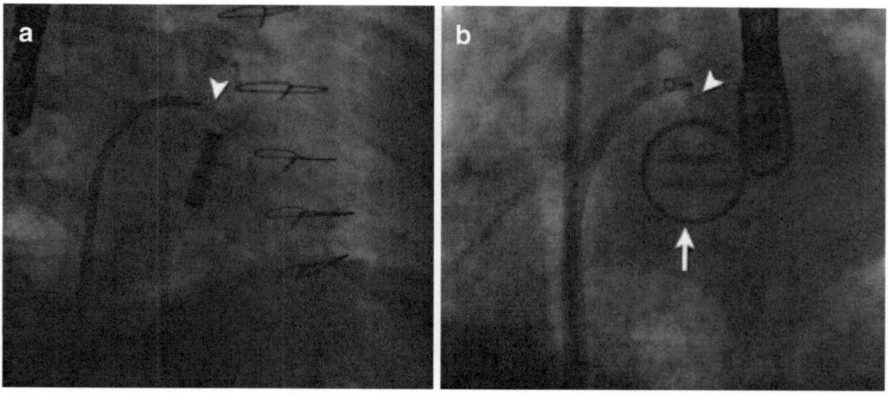

Fig. 5.6 Anterograde transseptal approach for para-mitral regurgitation. (**a**) Right anterior oblique (RAO) fluoroscopic projection of a steerable sheath and a mechanical mitral valve with leaflets open. A single *Amplatzer™ Vascular Plug II Occluder* (St Jude Medical Inc) is in position (*arrowhead*). (**b**) LAO–caudal fluoroscopic projection shows an *en-face* view of the same prosthetic mitral valve (*arrow*). Arrowhead again indicates the AVP II occluder

retrograde transapical approach was attempted (Videos 5.1, 5.2, 5.3, 5.4, 5.5, 5.6, and 5.7). On this occasion, implantation of the paravalvular leak closure device was successful leading to reduction in mitral regurgitation (Videos 5.8, 5.9, 5.10, 5.11, 5.12, and 5.13). The LV iatrogenic apical defect was closed using a coil. Post-procedure the patient remained hypotensive due to the development of haemothorax. Anticoagulation was not reversed due to the two mechanical valves being present. Emergency left thoracotomy was performed later that evening and the haematoma was evacuated. Despite the LV coil being undisplaced, the LV apex was noted to be bleeding and was therefore covered with pledgets. Post-operatively, the patient was managed on the Intensive Care Unit. Despite subsequent sepsis, she was successfully discharged on 28th January 2011 with a referral for consideration of surgical closure. Unfortunately, she continued to deteriorate in the community setting and died in 2012.

Para-aortic Valve Prosthesis Leak Closure

Most para-aortic defects can be approached retrogradely with TTE and fluoroscopic guidance. ICE is also very helpful when the probe is positioned in the right ventricular outflow tract just adjacent to a para-aortic defect. Because many of these defects are located anteriorly, the straight lateral fluoroscopic view is used with the right anterior oblique gantry positioned to provide an orthogonal view of the prosthesis.

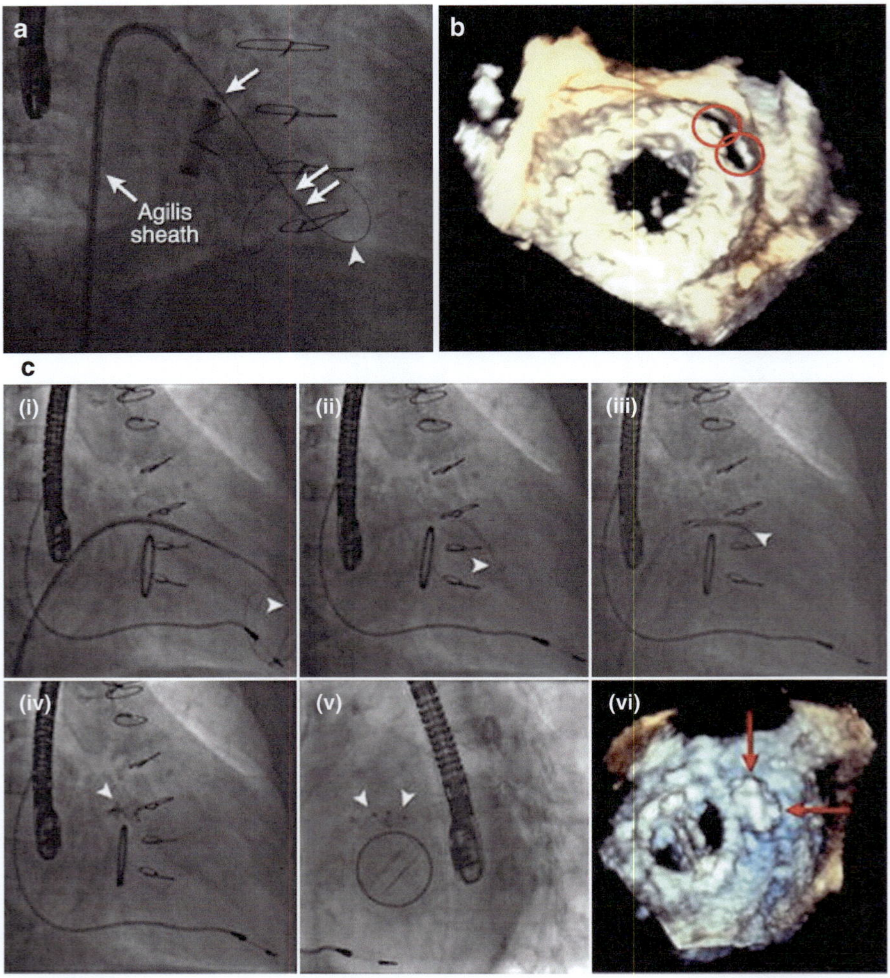

Fig. 5.7 Multiple sequential device deployment. (**a**) Telescoping coaxial catheter system. RAO view shows a left atrial steerable sheath (*Agilis™ NxT Steerable Introducer;* St. Jude Medical), a 6F 100 cm multipurpose coronary guiding catheter (*single arrow*), a 5F 125 cm multipurpose diagnostic catheter (*pair of arrows*) crossing the defect, and a stiff, angled glide wire (*arrowhead*) looped in the LV. (**b**) Device sizing for oblong defects. 3D TOE image of a mitral valve prosthesis shows an oblong defect. Successful closure of the defect with a single device requires a relatively large occluder, which increases the risk of prosthetic impingement due to device overhang. Closure with multiple smaller occluders (*circled in red*) can result in procedural success with a lower risk of prosthetic impingement. (**c**) Simultaneous device deployment technique. (**i**) Two 0.032-in wires are positioned across the paravalvular defect (*arrowhead*). (**ii**) Two separate 6 F multipurpose guide catheters are advanced across the defect (*arrowhead*). (**iii, iv**) Two *Amplatzer™ Vascular Plug II* devices are advanced and simultaneously positioned across the paravalvular defect (*arrowhead*). (**v**) LAO–caudal *en-face* view of the final device position, deployed side-by-side in the defect (*arrowheads*). (**vi**) Corresponding 3D TOE view of final device position (*red arrows*)

As with para-mitral defects, excellent visualisation of mechanical leaflets when present must be ensured.

Para-aortic defects are typically smaller than para-mitral defects and can usually be closed with a single device. If more than one device is judged to be likely, an anchor wire technique may be used, where a stiff guidewire is placed in the LV with a curve shaped to the ventricular size. Over this wire, an 8F Shuttle sheath can be placed and devices delivered sequentially as described for the treatment of para-mitral defects.

Coronary artery obstruction may occur when para-aortic defects are treated, because devices can protrude over coronary artery ostia. Numerous imaging planes may be necessary to demonstrate occlusion or clearance because two-dimensional fluoroscopic imaging can cause significant overlap between devices and ostia.

Case Study: Aortic Position

A 54 year old gentleman with severe aortic stenosis due to bicuspid aortic valve underwent aortic valve replacement (AVR) using a 21 mm Hancock Mosaic porcine bioprosthesis in 2010. Early para-aortic regurgitation was noted and the patient was referred for consideration of percutaneous leak closure in 2011 (Video 5.14, Fig. 5.8). No haemolysis or endocarditis was evident. LV function and dimensions were normal. Para-valvular closure was performed under general anaesthetic with peri-procedural TOE guidance using an *Amplatzer™ Vascular Plug III* closure device (AVP III, St Jude Medical Inc; Videos 5.15, 5.16, 5.17, 5.18, 5.19, and 5.20). The procedure was uncomplicated. Post-procedural TTE and TOE at 6 weeks and 6 months showed significant reduction in para-aortic valve leak and normal AVR function.

The Evidence Base for Para valvular Leak Closure

The largest series to date is of 141 defects that were closed in 115 patients (mean age: 67 ± 12 years; 53 % men). Most defects were para-mitral (78 %), with the remaining being para-aortic. Severe heart failure was present in 93 % of patients and some degree of haemolysis in 37 %. Nineteen patients had multiple treated defects. Snaring and wire exteriorisation was used in 29 patients (25 %); LV apical puncture was required in 13 cases. Devices were implanted in 125 defects (89 % of total defects) which is similar to that reported by Ruiz et al for 44 treated patients. Mean procedure time was 147 ± 54 min, but decreased with increasing experience. In 90 % of cases, regurgitation severity reduced considerably to 2+ or less; in 77 % of cases, severity was reduced to 1+. The authors reported several procedural failures early in their experience related to prosthetic leaflet impingement in 5 patients, and the inability to cross defects in 3 patients. Severe residual regurgitation persisted despite device placement in 11 patients. In 3 patients, devices had to be retrieved: one

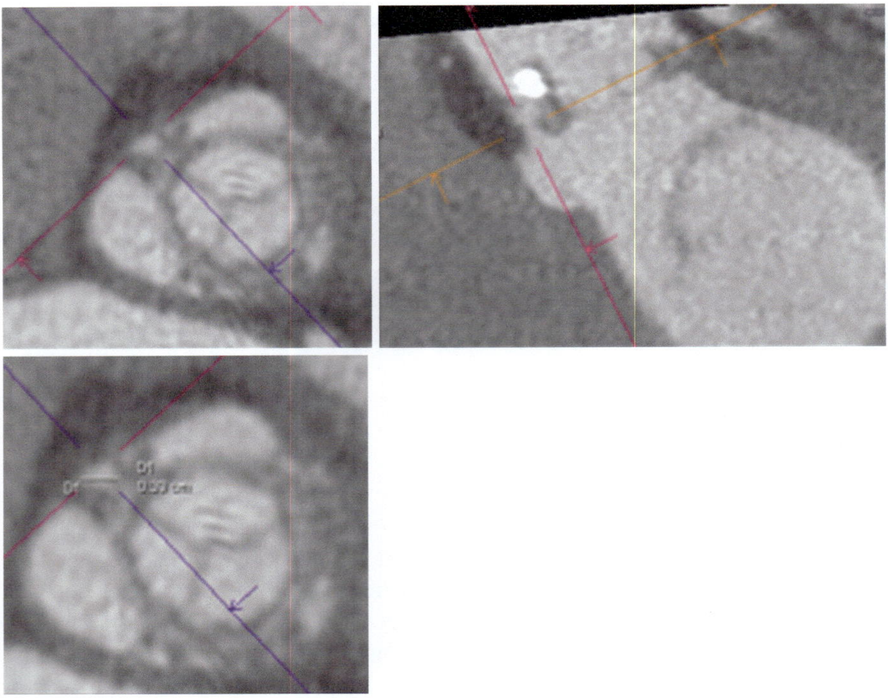

Fig. 5.8 Cardiac computed tomogram of aortic paravalvular leak demonstrating defect diameter and anatomy

device was mal-positioned in a prosthetic valve strut within the LV, and two embolized to the common iliac arteries. Total 30-day complication rate was 8.7 %. Complications included one sudden death 28 days after a successful procedure; one emergency surgery for prosthetic leaflet impingement; three strokes, including one related to transition of anticoagulation; two device embolisations without sequelae but necessitating retrieval; one unknown cause of death; and four hemothoraces after LV apical puncture. Of note, closure of apical puncture sites with vascular plugs or surgical glue has been utilised to help promote haemostasis. Similar types and incidence of complications were reported by Ruiz et al.

Procedural time, radiation dose, and technical results have improved with greater numbers of procedures performed. Importantly, acute technical success is a determinant of long-term outcome. In a study of 126 patients, 72 % of survivors were free of severe symptoms or need for surgery at 3-year follow-up. However, those with moderate or severe residual regurgitation had poorer survival free of death and severe symptoms (30.3 %) compared with those who had no (63.3 %) or mild (58.3 %) residual regurgitation ($p=0.01$). Moreover, symptom improvement occurred only in patients who had no or mild residual regurgitation. As expected in this high-risk population, non-cardiac morbidity was responsible for one-third to one-half of deaths at follow-up. Nevertheless, long-term clinical efficacy is highly dependent on residual regurgitation.

Future of Paravalvular Leak Closure

There will continue to be an increase in the need for paravalvular leak closure given the longevity of patient survival post-valve replacement. Closures will be required for individuals who have undergone TAVI – Transcatheter Aortic Valve Implantation. Access and expertise in advanced multimodality imaging techniques is vital in addition to experienced interventional operators, and this procedure will remain within regional tertiary centres.

Recommended Reading

1. Ruiz CE, Jelnin V, Kronzon I. Clinical outcomes in patients undergoing percutaneous closure of periprosthetic paravalvular leaks. J Am Coll Cardiol. 2011;58:2210–7.
2. Sorajja P, Cabalka AK, Hagler DJ, Rihal CS. Percutaneous repair of paravalvular prosthetic regurgitation: acute and 30-day outcomes in 115 patients. Circ Cardiovasc Interv. 2011;4: 314–21.
3. Sorajja P, Cabalka AK, Hagler DJ, Rihal CS. Long-term follow-up of percutaneous repair of paravalvular prosthetic regurgitation. J Am Coll Cardiol. 2011;58:2218–24.

Chapter 6
Percutaneous Closure of Patent Foramen Ovale (PFO)

Pradeep Magapu and Nick Palmer

Patent foreman ovale (PFO) is common in the adult population with a prevalence of 25 %. The foreman ovale is an anatomical structure that develops during foetal growth which allows passage of blood from the right into the left atrium. In utero, it allows blood to bypass the inactive pulmonary circulation (Fig. 6.1). At birth, there is a rapid fall in right heart pressures as the lungs expand, in addition to a rapid rise in left heart pressures, causing the foreman ovale to close. In a proportion of individuals, there is inadequate closure and a PFO is maintained. Unlike other atrial septal defects, PFO represents a 'flap' type defect that can remain clinically quiescent until such conditions exist to allow the flap to be opened. Important clinical situations which cause temporary or permanent increases in pulmonary artery pressures are coughing or pulmonary hypertension.

PFOs have been linked with several different conditions, cryptogenic cerebrovascular accidents (CVA) being the most reported. There are also suggested associations with decompression sickness (DCS), paradoxical embolization and migraine. The incidence of PFO in cryptogenic CVA is as high as 40 %, predominantly via paradoxical emboli, specifically thrombi from the venous circulation into the arterial circulation. Many people with PFO remain asymptomatic and the defect is found after specific investigations are undertaken to look for aetiology of a systemic complication. The most commonly employed imaging modality is transthoracic echocardiography (TTE) with agitated saline solution – "Bubble Contrast Echocardiogram". The defect can then be further investigated with transoesophageal echocardiography (TOE) and cardiovascular magnetic resonance (CMR) to further assess cardiac structure and calculate degree of shunt, avoiding the need for right heart catheterization.

Electronic supplementary material The online version of this chapter (doi:10.1007/978-1-4471-4981-1_6) contains supplementary material, which is available to authorized users.

P. Magapu (✉) • N. Palmer (✉)
Liverpool Heart and Chest Hospital, Liverpool, UK
e-mail: Pradeep.magapu@lhch.nhs.uk; pmagapu@hotmail.com; nick.palmer@lhch.nhs.uk

A. Varghese et al. (eds.), *Cases in Structural Cardiac Intervention*,
DOI 10.1007/978-1-4471-4981-1_6

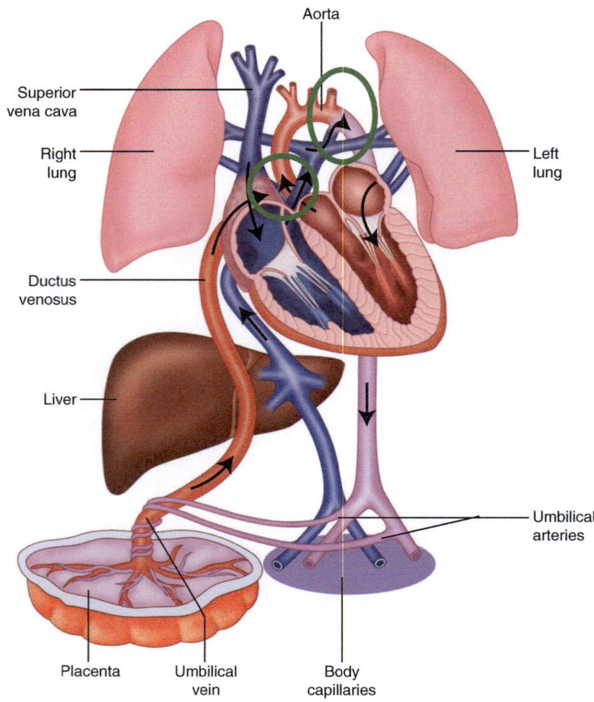

Fig. 6.1 Cartoon schematic of the foetal circulation. There are two shunts that provide shortcuts for most of the pulmonary circulation system (*circled in green*). Connection between the right and left atria via the foramen ovale. Connection between the truncus pulmonalis and the aorta via the ductus arteriosus

PFO defects can be closed surgically or using a percutaneous device. Due to the associated morbidity, surgical closure is chosen for individuals with other cardiac defects requiring operative intervention. One example of a percutaneous PFO closure device is the Amplatzer™ PFO Occluder (St Jude Medical Inc; Fig. 6.2). Other devices include the Amplatzer™ Septal Occluder (St Jude Medical Inc) and Helex® Septal Occluder (WL GORE, Newark, DE), which are predominantly used in atrial septal defect closure (Fig. 6.3).

Case Study

A 29 year old male was referred to our tertiary cardiac intervention centre for consideration of percutaneous PFO closure. His had presented to his local cardiology department with dizziness and headache in combination with right sided upper and lower limb weakness. Following a diagnosis of CVA, a series of investigations were undertaken to establish an aetiology. Routine haematological and biochemical investigations were unremarkable. Thrombophilia and auto-immune screens were negative. Computed tomography angiogram of his neck and cerebral vessels did not demonstrate dissection or other significant pathology. Brain magnetic resonance imaging (MRI) demonstrated multiple areas of infarction in the left posterior

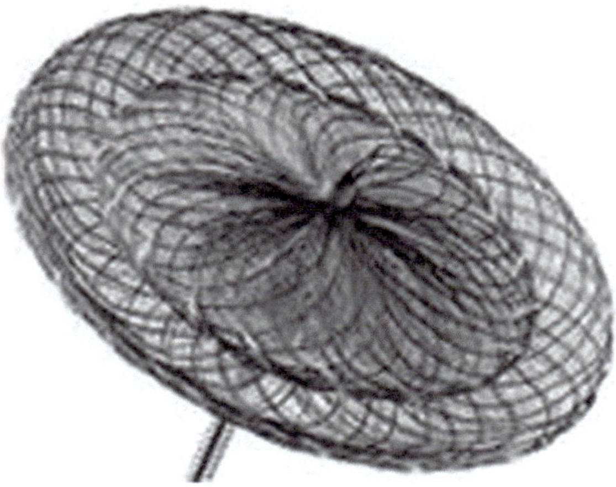

Fig. 6.2 St Jude Amplatzer™ PFO Occluder. This is a self-expandable, double disc device made from a nitinol wire mesh and thin polyester fabric. The two discs are linked together by a short, connecting waist which allows free motion of each disc (AMPLATZER and St. Jude Medical are trademarks of St. Jude Medical, Inc. or its related companies. Reproduced with permission of St. Jude Medical, © 2016. All rights reserved)

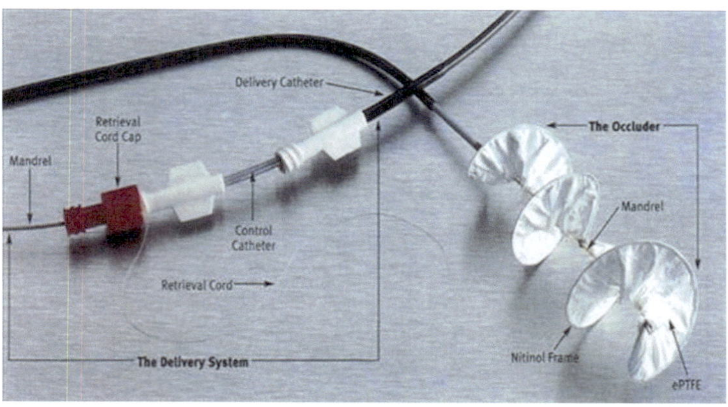

Fig. 6.3 Helex® Septal Occluder (WL GORE, Newark, DE). (**a**) Occluder and the delivery system. The occluder is designed as a single piece of ePTFE attached throughout its length to a nitinol frame wire. This leaves very little metal exposed to bloodstream (From *Circulation*. 2001;104: 711–6.)

cerebral artery territory. Twenty-four hour holter monitor recorded sinus rhythm throughout with no paroxysmal arrhythmia. A TTE study was undertaken, baseline images demonstrated an aneurysmal inter-atrial septum and bubble contrast echocardiography was performed. At rest, no bubbles were seen to cross the septum but following Valsalva, bubbles were clearly evident within the left atrium, suggestive of a clinically significant PFO.

PFO closure was performed under conscious sedation using a combination of midazolam and fentanyl with antibiotic and anticoagulant cover. Local anaesthetic was

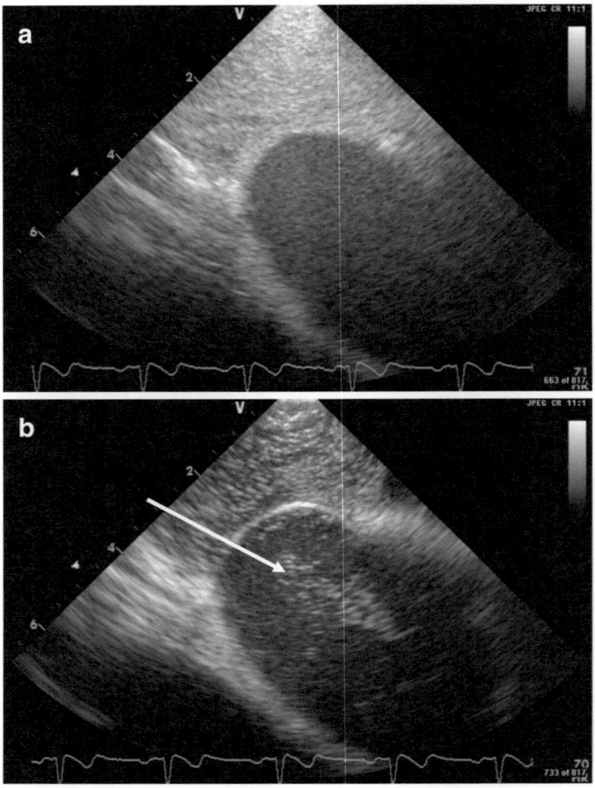

Fig. 6.4 Intracardiac echocardiogram (ICE). (**a**, **b**) ICE of positive bubble study with bubbles within the left atrium (*white arrow*)

administered to the right groin and sequential punctures of the femoral vein were performed. Two sheaths were inserted into the femoral vein (6 French [6 F] and 8 French [8 F]). Via the 6 F sheath, a multi-purpose A2 (MP-A2) catheters was passed on a standard length (150 cm) J tip wire. The 8 F sheath was used to pass an intracardiac echocardiogaphy (ICE) device up to the right atrium. With the ICE catheter in place, an on-table contrast study was performed, confirming the presence of an aneurysmal inter-atrial septum and septal defect following intermittent increases in right heart pressures (Video 6.1; Fig. 6.4a, b). The MP-A2 catheter was then used to cross the defect and cannulate the left upper pulmonary vein (Video 6.2; Fig. 6.5). Using a long exchange wire (260 cm straight tip) an 8 F TorqVue™ delivery system was placed in the left atrium. A 25 mm Amplatzer™ PFO Occluder was deployed into the left atrium and pulled into position under both echocardiography and fluoroscopy guidance (Video 6.3a, b; Fig. 6.6). Stability of the occluder was confirmed (Video 6.4 – Fluoroscopy) and once the operator was satisfied with its position, the device was released from the delivery shaft (Video 6.5 – Fluoroscopy). A final fluoroscopy image was acquired with the device in situ (Video 6.6; Fig. 6.7) and a final ICE image was obtained with colour flow Doppler across the occlusion device to demonstrate no residual shunt immediately post deployment (Video 6.7; Fig. 6.8). All the equipment was then removed and manual pressure was applied to achieve haemostasis.

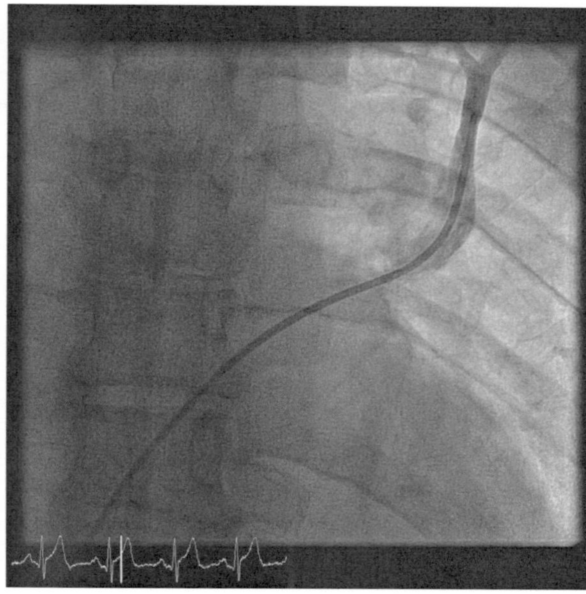

Fig. 6.5 Angiographic image of MP-A2 catheter positioned in left upper pulmonary vein

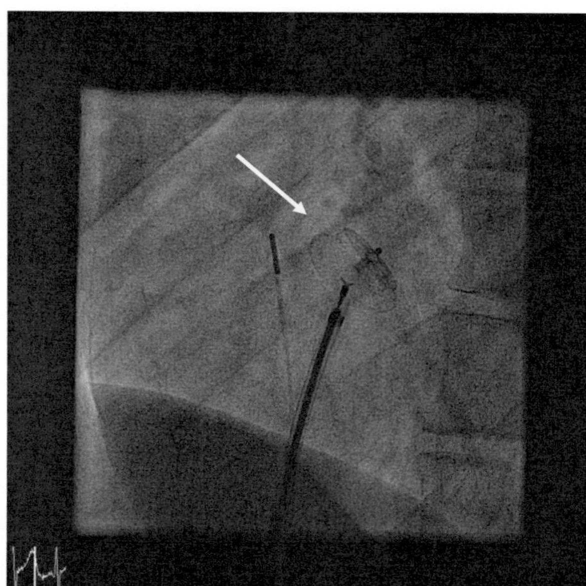

Fig. 6.6 Positioning of PFO occluder (*arrowed*)

The patient was transferred to the recovery area on the Day Ward for further monitoring. Targeted TTE was performed prior to discharge to confirm satisfactory and stable device position. No post procedural complications occurred and the patient was discharged home the same day.

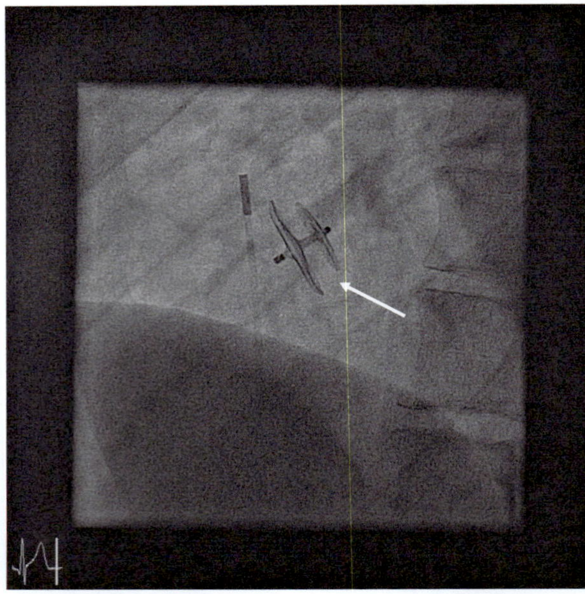

Fig. 6.7 Device *in-situ* (*arrowed*)

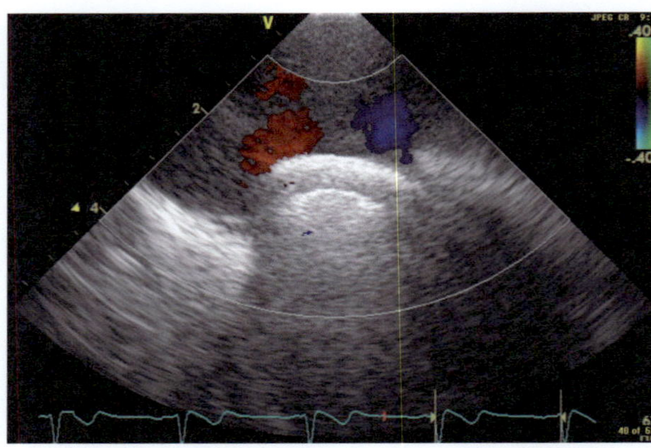

Fig. 6.8 Colourflow Doppler across occluder showing absence of inter-atrial shunt

Indications for PFO Closure

Indications for percutaneous PFO closure is an area of ongoing debate. The National Institute of Clinical Excellence (NICE) has provided three interventional procedure guidelines – IPG370, IPG371, IPG472.

Cryptogenic CVA

Treatment options for paradoxical embolization or systemic complications of PFO are pharmacological and/or closure of the defect. Three large randomised controlled trials have been undertaken to try and evaluate the benefits of percutaneous closure against medical therapy. Overall, they have demonstrated reduction in the incidence of CVA post closure compared to medical therapy alone. A meta-analysis of 58 observational studies with a pooled population of 10,327 subjects (8,185 PFO closure versus 2142 medical therapy) suggested an event rate of 0.8 % per 100 patient years in the closure group compared to 4.4 % per 100 patient years in the medical therapy group. Studies have also demonstrated that the procedure is well tolerated with low complication rates – risks are <0.1 %, 0.3 %, 0.1 %, 0.4 %, 0.4 %, 0.1 % for death, pericardial effusion, cardiac perforation, need for surgery, embolization of device, major bleed, air emboli, infective endocarditis and late thromboembolic disease, respectively. The main complication of percutaneous PFO closure remains atrial fibrillation (AF), which has been reported in up to 6 % of patients post device implantation. AF was transient in a small number.

Migraine

The use of percutaneous PFO closure devices in patients suffering from migraine is contentious and routine closure is not currently recommended. A cross-sectional study of subjects without evidence of CVA were screened using TTE to look for presence of a PFO. Within the cohort of individuals screened, migraine was noted in 16 %. In this study subset, incidence of PFO was 15 %. There was no significant difference in the finding of a PFO between subjects with or without migraine. A randomised controlled trial looking at the reduction in symptoms and headache days did not demonstrate any statistical difference between percutaneous PFO closure and a sham procedure. Both interventions were associated with an equal reduction in severity and duration of headaches.

NICE recommendation for the closure of a PFO in the treatment of migraine states that consultation with a Neurologist should be performed prior referral to an Interventional Cardiologist. Patients and carers must be counselled regarding the limited evidence of success in this field. Additionally, risks are still present, although low.

Divers and Decompression Sickness

The complication of acute DCS (also called the bends or caisson disease) is a valid concern amongst commercial and recreational divers caused by inadequate decompression following exposure to increased pressure. During a dive, the body tissues absorb nitrogen from the breathing gas in proportion to the surrounding pressure. If the diver remains at pressure, the gas presents no problem. When pressure is reduced too quickly, the nitrogen comes out of solution and forms bubbles in the tissues and bloodstream. This can lead to a myriad of symptoms including fatigue, joint pain, dyspnoea, numbness, tingling, and paralysis. In the presence of a PFO, transit of micro-bubbles from the venous circulation to the arterial circulation is allowed, bypassing the lungs where they would normally be filtered and increasing the risk of DCS.

PFO closure in this setting has not been investigated in a randomised controlled trial and only small cohort studies exist. Of 29 subjects who underwent PFO closure for DCS, 26 (79 %) returned to diving with no further episodes. Guidance from NICE states that there is still a risk involved with this procedure despite the high success rate of closure, and that patients should be fully informed of the risk versus benefits. Discussion should ideally be led by specialists in Diving Medicine prior to cardiology referral.

Future of Percutaneous PFO Closure

Evidence in favour of PFO closure is most widely available in the setting of cryptogenic CVA. More research is required in individuals at high risk as suggested either anatomically or with significant shunting. Evidence for closure in migraine remains scant and it is our opinion that this intervention should not be undertaken at the current time. In DCS, there is no evidence for pre-emptive PFO closure in asymptomatic divers. In the first instance altering dive techniques and practises may be as important as closing the PFO. Percutaneous PFO closure has high technical procedural success rates and low (rare) associated complications. Multi-disciplinary approach to patient selection is key with combined input as required from Stroke Physicians, Imaging and Interventional Cardiologists.

Recommended Reading

1. Percutaneous closure of patent foramen ovale to prevent recurrent cerebral embolic events – NICE interventional procedure guidance [IPG472] Published date: December 2013 http://www.nice.org.uk/guidance/ipg472.
2. Tobis J, Shenoda M. Percutaneous treatment of patent foramen ovale and atrial septal defects. J Am Coll Cardiol. 2012;60:1722–32.

Conclusion

Using a series of case studies, we have illustrated important percutaneous strategies to treat cardiac pathology that would previously have mandated cardiac surgery. These complex interventions will continue to increase as operator knowledge and expertise grows and technology advances. A wider role for these interventions will be driven further by an ageing patient population whose associated co-morbidities may preclude established surgical techniques as the optimal management option. Patient choice will also play a part with the increased awareness of minimally invasive strategies. Close collaboration between cardiologists with an interventional background and their colleagues with skills in advanced imaging will play a central role towards procedural success.

A. Varghese et al. (eds.), *Cases in Structural Cardiac Intervention*,
DOI 10.1007/978-1-4471-4981-1

MIX
Papier aus verantwortungsvollen Quellen
Paper from responsible sources
FSC® C105338

If you have any concerns about our products,
you can contact us on
ProductSafety@springernature.com

In case Publisher is established outside the EU,
the EU authorized representative is:
Springer Nature Customer Service Center GmbH
Europaplatz 3, 69115 Heidelberg, Germany

Printed by Libri Plureos GmbH
in Hamburg, Germany